A PEEP BEHIND THE SCREENS

(1940-1945)

by

Beryl S. Ozanne

A PEEP BEHIND THE SCREENS

ISBN 0 952 45790 3

Copyright   Beryl S. Ozanne

October 1994

Conditions of sale
This book is sold subject to the conditions that it shall not, by way of trade *or otherwise,* be lent, re-sold, hired out or otherwise circulated without the publisher's prior consent in any form of binding or cover other than that in which it is published *and without a similar condition including this condition being imposed on the subsequent purchaser.*

Copies of "A Peep behind the Screens" are available from
Beryl S. Ozanne, The Wing, Le Courtil Griffin,
Rue des Cottes, La Passee, St. Sampson's,
Guernsey, GY2 4TS
Tel. 01481 56704

Printed by The Guernsey Press Co. Ltd.,
Guernsey, Channel Islands.

I wish to dedicate this book to my family, with my love and many thanks for all their help and understanding.

A special thank you to two of my grand-daughters:
    Nicola Tomlins for designing the cover,
    Rebecca Breton for the illustrations.

Many thanks to Miss M.F. Collas, S.R.N., C.M.B., for her comments.

Not forgetting the help and advice I have received from Gwen and Rosaline, very many thanks to you both.

Beryl S. Ozanne

CONTENTS

	Page
Introduction	1
June 1940	3
The Last Friday in June 1940	5
Making their presence felt	11
Autumn 1940	13
Changes	22
Pillow Fight	23
The Unexpected	26
Life must go on	27
The Germans Intervened	30
Deportations	32
Malnutrition	33
Nurses' Billets	34
Cycles Everywhere	38
Hospital Way of Life	40
"Incidents"	46
Night Duty	50
Thrown in at the deep end	53
Forced Labourers	57
Radios Confiscated	58
Entertainment	60
Visiting Times	61
Anaesthetics	65
Life goes on	66
The Ward Cat	67
The Children's Ward	69
Theatre Work	75
Topic of Conversation	85
October 1943	88
Home Made Entertainment	88
I pray in the morning ...	102
Facing the Challenges	103
Christmas Carols	110
The Occupying Forces	115
Contents of Red Cross Parcels	120
Ghosts	122
Real Hunger	124
Guernsey, the isle of plenty	128
The Local "Press"	129
To our Canadians	142
The Evacuees Return	143
Getting Back to Normal	148

ILLUSTRATIONS

	Page
In St. John Ambulance Uniform	6
The States Emergency Hospital Buildings	15
"Please try and keep tidy for Matron's rounds"	18
"And what do you think you're doing"	24
Cottage where Nurses were billetted	34
"Lizzie"	44
Nurse Steiner	68
"Nursey, Nursey, can't see me!"	69
Group of Hospital Staff at time of Liberation	80
The theatre	81
The three patriots!	90
Christmas Morning Carols	109
Christmas Card	113
Liberation Card	132
Matron's at retirement, with two Sisters	132
The Mouse Trap	137
The Canadian St. John Ambulance Nurses	142

INTRODUCTION

This little account is a tribute to the wonderful work of those dedicated people who gave so much during the hard times.

Many years have passed since these happenings so it is impossible to recall everything in detail. I hope I am able to enlighten folk with these few facts.

It was my family who persuaded and encouraged me to write down a few little anecdotes of life at the States Emergency Hospital during the occupation.

You will note that, with a few exceptions, I have not mentioned names as I do not wish to embarrass or upset either ex-staff or ex-patients. Even though many of whom I have written have since passed on, there's bound to be either a relative or close friend who would have known them.

We were virtually a group of young local girls who were trained and guided by the staunch and dedicated work of the Doctors, Matrons, Sisters and Staff Nurses who stayed behind to keep the Medical Services of the island going through those traumatic years. So many people owe so much to those who so willingly chose to stay and serve the islanders who had remained in Guernsey.

The Doctors were fantastic. There was no popping over the water to catch up on all the latest skills and medication. They all worked as a team to the very best of their joint abilities and whatever medications that were available.

I sincerely hope I have not given the impression that it was all fun and games with lots of laughter. Nothing could be further from the truth, though I have tried to convey the lighter side of things.

We were literally cut off from the rest of the world. Every man, woman and child just <u>had</u> to make the best of things.

I should like to pay tribute to the members and staff of the St. John Ambulance Brigade who supported us all through that time. They did a wonderful job for the islanders.

JUNE 1940

The busy little island of Guernsey in the height of the tomato season.

Of course we knew there was a war on and many of the island's young men and women were serving in H.M. Forces. Every day, with pride, we'd read in our daily "Press" about our own kith and kin doing their bit for King and Country.

We considered ourselves very lucky to be living in such a beautiful environment: still able, more or less, to continue as usual. The shipping of goods to and from the U.K. carried on. We had H.M. Army protecting us. There were a few manned anti-aircraft guns at strategic points. We were O.K.!

Then, suddenly, the Army and guns were withdrawn and we were an "Open Town" - "So what?" - No one was going to bother about little Guernsey, least of all "Jerry".

The next we knew, was, all the schools were to be evacuated to the mainland. The population was in a turmoil. The quiet living, contented Guernseyman didn't know which way to turn or what to do for the best.

With only a few hours' notice, the school children began to embark, their teachers and a few voluntary helpers accompanying them. No one seemed to know _why_ there was all this upheaval.

Parents had hastily packed a change of clothing, plus food for the journey, hoping they were doing the right thing for their children _and_ that they would see them again in the very near future.

It was known by then that evacuation was voluntary, but a lot of people had already decided to go. Some mothers went with their children, leaving father behind to sort things out and then hope to meet up with the family in the U.K. later - or the father left to go and serve in the forces, thinking that the wife and children would be better to stay put. And, of course, many children went away leaving both their parents behind.

Many islanders just rushed off leaving everything, taking just what they could carry in the way of clothing.

It was a pitiful sight to see cattle, chickens, tame rabbits, goats, caged-birds all set free and left to fend for themselves, just strolling about lost and unhappy; the poor cattle waiting to be milked. Thankfully, those farmers left on the island rallied round and looked after all the animals.

We, my immediate family, decided to leave the island, but wished, if possible, to sail out to New Zealand to join the family out there. We were awaiting confirmation of bookings on a liner due to leave the U.K. within 2-3 days – we waited for a very long time!

The following week things changed again. Ships were leaving loaded with tomatoes once more and making for the U.K. Things seemed to be more settled.

All around the island were posters stating "No place like home!" "Why go mad!" "Don't be Yellow!"

And folk began to relax, hoping for the best. After all we were "An Open Town"!

BUT:

There was evidence of something sinister in the air – we didn't take a lot of notice, but the fact that there were high-flying aircraft about quite frequently made us wonder just what was happening on the nearby coast of France.

Now and then a 'plane would fly lower; "reconnaissance planes". Then we realized that they were German 'planes and we got quite used to seeing a Swastika now and then. Little did we guess what was to happen within the next couple of days.

THE LAST FRIDAY IN JUNE 1940
LATE AFTERNOON

It had been a really beautiful day – then shock and horror.

On the White Rock (the harbour) there was the usual stream of lorries laden with chip-baskets of tomatoes for the U.K. Lorry drivers awaiting their turn to ship their lorry load and then get back home for their evening meal with the family. When – there was a terrible roar as five German bombers swooped in from over the sea, attacked the docks, the ships, civilians and the whole line of lorries which extended up as far as the Weighbridge. Not satisfied with the bombing, they flew all along the jetty machine-gunning everything and everyone in sight – what carnage – what destruction within minutes!

At the time I was living at my home in St. Martin's with my father (my mother having passed away a few months earlier). I could hear the terrible explosions and machine-gun fire and could see great clouds of black smoke billowing over the town and harbour area and 'planes circling overhead.

A neighbour and I just stood and watched "dumbfounded". He suddenly cried "Look at that! The "so and so's" are bombing us!"

I suddenly pulled myself together. This is what we had been training for, all those past weeks at the First Aid and A.R.P. Station. Training just in case there ever was a raid.

I collected my tin-hat, gas-mask, first aid kit and the trusty old cycle, then made for the First Aid Post, which was at the St. Martin's Parish Hall (a 10-minute ride).

On the way no one was in sight. I don't know what had happened to everyone, except, that is, one bus driver who had pulled his bus in under some trees at the roadside. He had crawled under the bus and was absolutely terrified, he shouted to me to join him in his shelter, but I explained to him, I just <u>had</u> to get on duty. After checking that he'd be O.K. I went on my way. I must say I was quite apprehensive and did try to take cover as I went, as 'planes were still buzzing around and there was the sound of bursts from machine-guns.

The caretaker at the "Post" was busy stoking up the boiler and we were the only two there for quite a time, during which we prepared the receiving area, in case any casualties appeared. Then other members began to arrive and we soon had everything ready.

Little by little we got news of the terrible happenings at the harbour and were ordered to "stand by". A few people, shocked and with minor injuries, did call in for treatment.

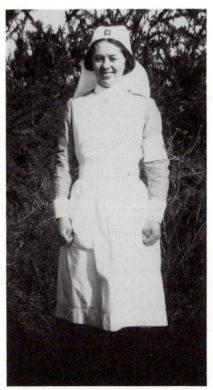 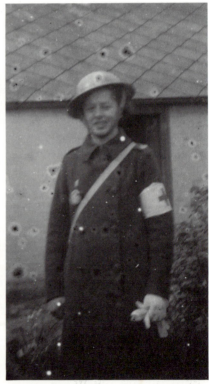

In St. John Ambulance Uniform

We were all on 'pins' waiting and wondering what would happen next. Eventually quite late in the evening a group of us were sent off in our lorry. We had been trained in groups and had been out on practice attending various incidents to treat "casualties" of mock raids and gas attacks. But – this was for real.

Our team set off heading for the harbour. Up until then, things had not really hit me, but, sitting in the back of that lorry with colleagues among stretchers and all sorts of First Aid Equipment, I wondered what we were going to find!

My father at that time was running a tomato packing store in an area quite close to the harbour. He often drove a lorry-load of tomatoes down to the boat for shipping. He had several women packing the tomatoes at the store. How were they all, was everything alright? Was my father looking after them all? Or was he on the docks at the time of the bombing? I also had a brother-in-law who was a lorry driver for a different company. Was he O.K.? It didn't bear thinking about.

We were already passing the Town Church, everywhere we looked there was damage. Our lorry wheels were crunching through all the glass which had been blown out of the windows all along the front. The lovely old Town Church hadn't escaped, some of the beautiful church windows had been damaged too. There was glass and rubble everywhere.

Smoke was still billowing over the harbour. The Weighbridge too was badly damaged. The site of what had been a row of lorries waiting to ship their loads was just a lot of twisted iron and burning rubber; tomatoes squashed and pouring out of their containers didn't help the sight. It made one think of the blood of those hard working men that had been spilt and of those who most surely had perished that day. There was nothing for us to do there, so we made our way to the headquarters at the Town Arsenal.

Another sad sight met us as we drove up the Avenue. There, at the top was a St. John Ambulance at the side of the street riddled with bullet holes. We heard later that the

Ambulance had been attacked as it was driving off the harbour and was followed up the Avenue. The driver was killed and one of the officers in attendance was injured when he threw himself over the casualty who was on the stretcher. The St. John Ambulance man received some nasty wounds from which, fortunately, he made a full recovery. He had certainly saved the life of the casualty who was on that stretcher.

So many acts of bravery and courage were carried out that day, so many an unsung hero of whom we'll never hear.

We arrived at Headquarters, where we helped out with a few minor injuries. The majority had been dealt with earlier and the more serious cases transferred out to the Emergency Hospital where surgeons and staff worked through the night.

Back we went to St. Martin's to report that everything now appeared to be quiet. We cleared up our station carefully in case there would be another raid.

Many were the experiences we heard of that night and everyone was very tired. We set off for our homes, hoping we'd have a quiet night and hardly daring to think of what might happen next.

As I cycled home I worried as to what I'd find. Would my father be there? Had he been involved in the raid? Was he alive or injured? Were some of those twisted girders I'd seen part of his lorry? We had learnt during the course of the evening that some of the drivers had sheltered <u>under</u> the lorries, thinking they'd be safe, pour souls.

Riding around the back of my home, my heart in my mouth, what did I see? Thank God; I was so relieved to see a chink of light through the black-out in the kitchen window. I rushed in and was so thankful to see my father there, safe and sound. He, too, was grateful to see me safely returned.

He had been in the store at the time of the raid and had had a very stressful time trying to keep the women packers as safe and as calm as possible. Naturally they were all terrified and worried.

When it was quiet and the bombing etc. over, my father took them all in the lorry to their own homes, making sure they were all safe and sound before making his own way home. He knew that I had gone on duty, but of course worried as to where I was and what I was doing. We had so much to tell each other, and spent quite a time discussing all the happenings of the day.

Neither of us wanted to go to bed for fear of what might happen next. So, we spent the night in armchairs, fully dressed and with an overnight bag each packed and standing nearby.

The next couple of days were spent trying to decide what was the best thing to do. We were very fortunate that none of the family were injured, but, my brother-in-law will never ever forget that day. He had parked his vehicle in the line of lorries near the Weighbridge and had just got out of his lorry when he heard, and then saw, German 'planes swooping in over the docks. He just took to his heels and ran for his life toward the Sarnia sheds, in the Lower Pollet, and on looking back, all he saw where he'd left his lorry was twisted metal and some wheels.

All the family met up at my grandparents' home. We had all gone to check that they were alright. As we didn't all have 'phones we found that it was best to get together. Any family crisis seemed to lure us there.

So there we all were, plus my brother-in-law's parents, who were too nervous to be left on their own. What an upheaval, no one knew what was going to happen or what we should do next.

We all stayed over and spent another night fully dressed in arm-chairs or lying on the floor in blankets, no one wanted to go upstairs. Thank goodness Guernsey farm houses have spacious rooms.

No one knew <u>what</u> to expect and we were still all together on the Sunday, when suddenly a siren sounded, followed by the sound of 'planes' engines, but, no bombing. All was quiet for a while. Then the 'phone rang. It was friends who lived near the airport to say that two German 'planes had landed on our airport and men had been seen walking around before taking off again.

The same evening the sirens went off once more; 'planes were overhead going round and round, but no bombing, or firing. We just waited and waited in agonizing suspense, then at about 11 p.m. the "All Clear" sounded.

The buzzing of the engines had long ceased. We knew, yet dreaded to admit it. The island was <u>occupied</u> and we were <u>trapped</u>.

Another night of us all huddled under blankets. The thoughts that went through our minds! What would happen to us? What would we have to face up to? Would the men be taken away? Would we have to part with money and valuables? What would they do to the women? Questions and more questions! But no answers as yet.

Though we passed a sleepless night, at least it was uneventful.

Monday's local newspaper was full of orders.

We were occupied. Orders forbidding the use of vehicles, or any form of transport on the roads. All weapons had to be handed in at the Town Arsenal immediately and any members of H.M. Forces over here on leave had to give themselves up.

The days that followed were filled with the sound of aircraft engines of all types and sizes, hedge-hopping and skimming the roof-tops, doing as much as possible to un-nerve the population and terrify the already anxious islanders.

The huge troop carriers were so massive (the islanders christened them the "Black Pigs"). We had never seen such large aircraft.

German Forces were continually patrolling the island in commandeered cars, with much show of weapons and fixed bayonets.

Gradually the island settled down. We accepted our lot and tried to make the best of it.

I must say the first sight of German troops was somewhat daunting, but thank goodness they didn't bother us, and as time went by we just ignored them as much as possible.

The troops had been made to believe that they had landed in England. No amount of arguing would make them believe otherwise. I suppose the fact that we were English spoken convinced them that they were in England!

MAKING THEIR PRESENCE FELT

One early incident I remember well was in a town shop at the beginning of the occupation. It was in a hairdressers in the High Street which had a perfumery department.

Two officers marched in, of course they had to be served straightaway. When they came to pay for their goods they handed over German money. The proprietor was most indignant. He said, "I want proper money" – "That is proper money and the sooner you accept it as such the better. You just have to put up with it."

"But I don't understand the value of your money." – "Well, you're going to have to learn all about it, aren't you? Because we're not using English money and nor will you!"

The officer was a huge chap and the shop owner was a little French man with a black pointed beard. He was furious. I thought he'd have a heart attack. The other customers and myself wondered if we ought to make ourselves scarce or stop and watch the proceedings.

Another assistant came to serve us, while the Germans gave the Frenchman a lesson in German currency. After all these years I can still see the disgust and hatred on that Frenchman's face. I really feared for him at the time, but I think they forgave him, but made sure he knew who was "boss". They were very fluent in English. No doubt one of the reasons why they were in the island.

Progress was very slow. So many new laws, so much more rationing, the rations getting smaller as time went by.

The whole labour force was at sixes and sevens. The main industry of growing, picking, packing, carting and shipping tomatoes, had suddenly ceased and all delivery vans were off the road, unless of course they were taken over by the Germans.

Rumour had it that all men out of work were to be deported to France; so, anyone who had work that needed doing was good enough to employ one of his fellow islanders rather than see them go away. However, once again, it was just rumour.

The threat of men having to be deported would come up time and time again in the future. Many an alarming tale would be told as to what would happen to us if anyone dared to go against the German orders. We were just kept in constant dread of what <u>might</u> happen.

We gradually became accustomed to life under German rule and eventually felt we could laugh at many of the tales that were told rather than repeat them.

Everyone tried to settle to the new way of life and make the best of it all, though it was difficult. Every day the local Press was full of new rules and orders. This was *"verboten"* and that was *"verboten"*. Some of the orders we could just laugh at and some we had to just grin and bear.

Many islanders were employed by the Germans, a lot of folk didn't like the idea, but really had no choice.

However, it takes a lot to get a "True Guernsey Donkey" down, plus the fact that they can be extremely tolerant and able to keep tight-lipped when needs be.

It was a matter of just living day for day.

AUTUMNN 1940

In the autumn of 1940 I was approached by the Lady Superintendent of the St. John Ambulance Brigade, asking if I had ever considered taking up nursing. I had been a voluntary member of the St. John Ambulance for some time.

My reply to the query was that I didn't think myself capable of full-time nursing. However after quite a lot of persuading and assurance, I agreed to an interview with the Matron of the surgical wards at the Emergency Hospital. Suffice to say I was accepted or I wouldn't be writing this.

I feel a little explaining is needed here with regards to The Emergency Hospital, in the Câtel parish.

Before the second world war, we had the St. Peter Port Hospital (known as the Town Hospital) capably run by Matron B. and her staff, and throughout the occupation as a general hospital, but mostly for geriatric and long stay patients.

There were also two or three private Nursing Homes, and a Maternity Home known as the Lady Ozanne's Maternity Hospital at Cordier Hill in St. Peter Port, with Matron F. and her staff.

The Victoria Cottage Hospital, situated at Amherst, was under the supervision of Matron H. and her staff.

Then there was The Country Hospital at the Câtel, a general hospital, with Matron R. and her staff. This was the place that was chosen to house three hospitals under one roof for the duration of the war.

A vast building; the first floor was used as surgical wards with Matron H. and her staff. Second floor was for the medical cases supervised by Matron R. and her staff. The Maternity Ward was also on the second floor with the labour wards above. This was in charge of Matron F. and her staff. There was also an annexe where male mentally ill were cared for.

Originally The Country Hospital was self-supporting, with a farm, many outbuildings and very large gardens, plus fields surrounding this. There were several "inmates" who worked on the farm and in the gardens, also some helped in the kitchens and some with general cleaning.

At the beginning of the occupation the farm and garden produce was a great asset. But sadly the time came when there wasn't enough food for the animals. Fruit and vegetables had a habit of disappearing so, unfortunately, the hospital could no longer be self-supporting. However, with help from the "powers that be", whose job must have been very frustrating, The Emergency Hospital kept going.

Having the staffs of three hospitals to house became a problem. The original staff were already accommodated, but all the extra people needed to be housed, nursing staffs mostly and some domestics. Domestics either lived at home and came in daily, or were found accommodation at the hospital.

Across the fields behind The Emergency Hospital, on a hill, was the Children's Home, which had been evacuated and was standing empty. So the "powers that be" had a bright idea to house the overflow of nurses up there. That's where the Surgical and some Maternity Staffs were placed. We had no need to walk on the roads on our way on and off duty, as there was a pathway through the gardens and fields up to the Home. We were all issued with night-passes, so although there was a curfew, we were O.K.

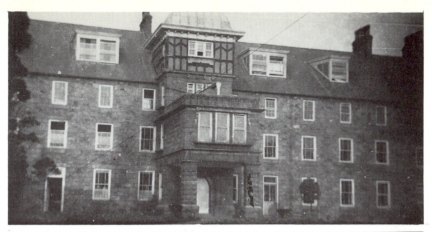

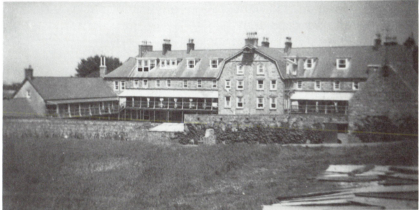

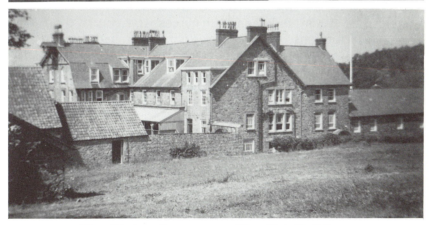

The States Emergency Hospital Buildings

There were two dormitories plus other single rooms. The dormitory I was in had six beds, with little three drawer dressing tables with mirrors, placed back to back between the beds, creating some sort of privacy, three beds each side of the room. There was a very large communal wardrobe at the far end. Twelve of us shared a bathroom in which there were two baths and four wash-hand basins, low set in the walls as they had been installed for children's use.

Can you imagine the bustle to get washed and dressed first thing in the morning, most of us half asleep and some not at their best at that time of the day? Fingers were all thumbs as we struggled with stiff collars, belts and cuffs and studs that just seemed to want to go anywhere but where they should; starched caps that had to be on just right and aprons that rustled every time you moved.

There was a general dash down the garden, up the flights of concrete stairways into the hospital. Then on to the ward to report to Sister, just in time!

After report a quick change of stiff cuffs for sleeve frills pulled neatly over the rolled-up sleeves, then paired off with another Nurse and a bright and brisk "Good morning" to the patients.

The day had started, up to 34 beds (when full) to be made up by 8 a.m. between four nurses. Of course there were many interruptions during the course of bed-making, the patient would often need something or other and often there'd be a patient who couldn't or just wouldn't co-operate.

My first duties were on men's surgical wards.

I felt a bit strange at first, but found the training I'd had with the St. John Ambulance and Nursing Division stood me in very good stead. I did know how to make a bed, hospital corners and all, and was quite well acquainted with hospital jargon, which was very handy.

I did enjoy working on that ward. The patients were a great bunch of lads. There were still a couple of men who had been injured in the raid. They were improving, albeit, slowly. Also there were three who had fallen from the St. Martin's Water Tower, they too were well on the road to recovery, and certainly played up to the nurses, all in good fun.

The nurse I was working with (senior to me) was short and rather plump, while I was tall and skinny, so of course these lads christened us Laurel and Hardy. Never could we walk the ward without the famous signature tune being whistled by at least half a dozen men. They were mostly fracture cases, so didn't feel sick and we had lots of teasing and cheek. However they didn't always get the better of the Nurses, far from it. They got as good as they gave.

Bed-making was always a problem on men's ward, with some, almost a fight. What man likes to be disturbed and made to look neat and tidy; we took all the moans and groans with good heart, but were always most careful and considerate not to make things too uncomfortable for those really ill.

There are many ways of making a bed. The rubber sheeting was the most objectionable thing; a large sheet covering the mattress, the bottom cotton sheet, another smaller rubber sheet covered with a cotton draw sheet, which, had there been a slight accident, could be easily changed. There's so many ways of making a bed, some are quite difficult but it is surprising how quickly one learns to cope with the varied cases, be it fractured limbs, abdominal operations etc. etc., to say nothing of those incontinent.

With patient comfortable against the pillows, then came the top sheet and blankets, top blanket bright red, then the white counterpane for day time, all smoothed down to perfection, corners just so and making sure that the openings of the pillow slips were turned away from the door, so that everything looked just perfect for Matron's rounds, not forgetting the bed ends in a straight line with wheels turned in and lockers neat and tidy.

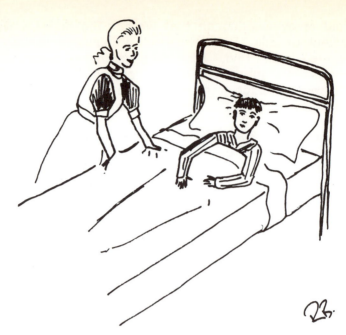

"<u>Please</u> try and keep tidy for Matron's rounds!"

One patient, on enquiring why the pillows had to be placed with openings away from the door, was promptly told by one Nurse "Oh! that's so that you don't get ear-ache with the draught from the door"!

At night, the white counterpanes were removed, folded and hung at the foot of the beds. This, in the half light of night gave a beautiful cosy look to the ward, with the glow of the red blankets against the white linen.

On day duty, once the beds were made it was time for Nurses' breakfast (two shifts for all meals) just half an hour in the dining-room then it was back to a hundred and one jobs. Bottle or Bed-pan rounds, cleaning sluices, arranging flowers, making sure they go to the right patient or there's trouble! Water glasses filled, Intakes and Outputs checked, then it's time for hot drinks, to say nothing of the dressings, hot fomentations and many other treatments. Another quick check that all the ward is spick and span, Matron's due on her rounds. There's a hush in the ward as she goes from bed to bed. Juniors just make themselves scarce, either in the sluice or anti-rooms, working at whatever is needed. Laying trays for dressings, making swabs and dressings ready for the drums which have to be sterilized - cleaning anything and everything in sight.

Then the Doctors start their ward visits and before we know it it's time to prepare the patients' dinner trays, then we juniors have to go right down to the kitchens and queue up to collect a very large tray, five dinner plates of food on each, to be carried up two flights of stairs, then taken around the ward to each patient as quickly as possible, before the food got cold. - No heated plates or cupboards or even porters to carry in those days. - We certainly got to know those stairs well.

(There came a time when this was greatly improved - each ward received sufficient dinners in large dishes i.e. one with potatoes, one veg, one meat or whatever, which were brought up from the kitchen by porter and male nurses and served on to plates by Sister in charge of ward. A much more sensible idea and more economical as each individual received what he could eat, no wastages on plates.)

On the ward, some were on special diets, some were unable to feed themselves, like the man who was unfortunate enough to break both his arms, when felling trees. - Another dash round to clear all trays and dishes and mop up any spills.

At last, time for our dinner, how great to be able to sit for half an hour. In the dining-room was one large long table. Here we'd meet our colleagues from the medical and maternity wards. What a lot of chat! All comparing different cases and exchanging some very humorous stories. Chat of off-duty activities and talk of our life under the German rule. - But - we had forgotten the saying that "walls have ears" and suddenly realized we'd have to be more careful in future as our dining-room maids were German girls who had been working in the island before the war as "au-pairs" and had been interned until the Germans took over and the internees were released. Many of them worked as domestics in the hospital.

From then on we were careful as to what we discussed in the dining-room, for fear of it being repeated to the authorities. This didn't stop us gossiping in the recreation room, though we were careful and always on the alert in case of eavesdroppers.

Afternoon ward duties in the main comprised bed-baths, treatments, and attending to teas. On visiting days we'd either do door duties, showing visitors in and answering their enquiries, or, we'd be tucked away out of sight preparing dressings, etc. until it was time to do the patients' teas.

If one was lucky enough to be on early tea-time (staff) we'd come back on the ward and find all patients' teas cleared and the next job was handing round all the washing bowls to those capable of washing themselves and washing those unable to cope on their own. Then all the backs to be rubbed, plus bottles and pans when needed, and temperatures to be taken and charted.

Doing backs was a job and a half in those days, giving a good rub with soap and water to all pressure points, then a dollop of methylated spirits, finished off with a good sprinkling of talcum powder. Patient all fresh and clean again (till the next time!).

Before you know it, it's patients' supper time; another rush around. Then staffs' supper-time. The day is nearly done.

Back on the ward after our supper, to attend to the patients again, beds straightened, pillows plumped up. Tooth mugs issued and teeth put to soak, hot-water bottles to fill. Tuck-up for the night all round and then: "Good night, everyone!" And hand over to the night staff. Report to Sister. "You may go Nurse." Music to the ears, what bliss. A quick bath, if you're lucky, only 4" water allowed, hot water rationed. Often no bath and wash down had to do. Then - bed, beautiful bed. What a day! My poor feet!

Still it's a real worthwhile job; wouldn't change it, in spite of all the hard slog.

A grateful smile from a patient for the smallest task, or, to see a patient leaving the ward feeling so much better than when they were admitted, and know that you have helped in some small way, makes it all worthwhile. It's a great life!

― ― ― ― ― ―

A rather amusing incident happened which gave me the opportunity of being employed at the hospital.

Apparently one of the older nurses who had been a V.A.D. during the 1914-18 war, had met with an accident. Whilst bed-making one day, she had dropped a chair on her foot and fractured her big toe. From then on she was known as Calamity Jane.

I had the pleasure of working with her, when she was fit again. She was a dear person, very dedicated, but so much older than the majority of the staff and I'm sorry to say, we were often amused by her old-fashioned ways and sayings.

I was rather mystified one day on her asking me to fetch the "Canterbury" from the sluice room. I just couldn't think what she meant, but making my way to the sluice room and thinking about what she was doing, and what she could possibly need, it suddenly dawned on me. What she wanted was a "Winchester" of disinfectant. A large glass bottle.

There were many very interesting characters amongst the patients, some of them long stay patients.

Captain, who was a retired Canadian Mountie, comes to mind. He was a somewhat crusty old chap at times, but, on his good days, he had many a story to tell, though he was a very modest man and was respected by all.

At times he was well enough to take a walk in the gardens and around the hospital farm, where he would spend some time with the gardeners and farm workers. This was at the beginning of the occupation.

When potatoes were plentiful he'd place two nice sized ones in the duty room Aga to warm while he got dressed, then he'd place one in each pocket of his jacket to keep him warm during his little walks.

I must explain; he was a far from well man and had no home over here; like many others he had become trapped on the island and owing to his illness had been unable to leave at the time of the evacuation. So, the hospital became his home and his few possessions in the ward with him. Had he been a fitter man he would no doubt have been deported like many others.

We were all very sad when Captain died and missed him a great deal.

CHANGES

Guernsey was changing rapidly in appearance and atmosphere. Everywhere one went we were sure to see German troops about, setting up various stations for their needs, taking over whatever took their fancy, irrespective of whose property it was, or what it was normally used for. If "Jerry" wanted it, he took it. They commandeered homes, folk were turned out at virtually a minute's notice.

Orders continued to be issued every day as to what the islanders could or could not do.

We soon got used to traffic driving on the right hand side of the road, not without a few accidents at first. Getting indoors before curfew was a bit of a bind at first, but we soon got used to it.

The town shops were looking rather sparse and troops bought up whatever took their fancy and paid for it with their paper money, which was another thing we had to learn about. Some shop-owners got wise after a bit and took a risk, when they could, of keeping some goods "under the counter" for the islanders. But they had to be very careful not to be caught, as there was fear of reprisals and sad to say, yes, there were some informers about.

Many officers paraded about, chests full of medals, very big fellows, no doubt sent over to put fear into the islanders. How we disliked them. Little did they know how tough the Guernseyman can be. In time we came to laugh at them behind their backs.

It was very demeaning, having these men telling us what to do, in our homes and all over our island.

PILLOW FIGHTS

As you can imagine, things were changing around the hospital too, and with the staff.

Being billeted at the Children's Home was quite fun, we were a happy crowd there. With curfew being from 9 p.m. to 6.30 a.m. meant quite long evenings with little to do.

In spite of all the hard work on the wards, we found ways of relaxing and "letting our hair down"!

Our dormitory had a stable door (it must have been for small children). As you can imagine the occupants of the other dormitory took full advantage. We were frequently "moo-ed" at and ribbed about animal habits and goodness knows what. We took it all in good part until someone suggested it was time we retaliated. We'd put up with their cheek and their jokes long enough.

One night, after lights out, six of us crept out of bed and clad in pyjamas with a pillow tucked under each arm, emerged one behind the other, feeling along the wall of the corridor, "shushing" each other as we went. Everything was well "blacked out".

We were just "creeping" along when, suddenly, there was a blaze of light. We did feel foolish. There was Sister, all stiff and starch and very poker faced.

"And what do you lot think you're doing after lights out?"

We felt and must have looked like a lot of silly little schoolgirls. Our spokesman, or should I say spokeswoman, the first in the line, said in a small voice:

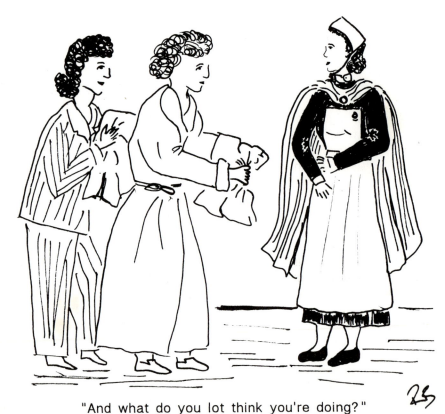

"And what do you lot think you're doing?"

"Sorry, Sister, we were just going to the other dormitory to pay them out for all their 'ragging'"

Still very poker faced, back came a sharp reply:

"I'm not stopping you! Go ahead and give it to them! But don't make a night of it. You Nurses have to be on duty early in the morning, you know. 'Good Luck' and don't make too much noise!"

We didn't need a second bidding. We all whispered. "Thanks Sister" and continued on our mission.

What a great fight. We certainly surprised that lot of sleeping beauties and had a great time, finishing up out in the corridor the lot of us, until, the lights went on again.

"Alright girls, that's enough. Lights out. Good Night." Sister again. What a good sport she was.

I must say that was the first of many "set to's" with the rival dormitory.

Another night they crept in on us and tipped us all out of our beds, literally. We awoke to find a nurse each end of our beds and they just tilted the beds rolling us out, legs and arms flying, mattresses and blankets all over the floor.

We had a good laugh trying to sort each other out and making up our beds again, all in the dark of course, and with a lot of giggling and whispering.

I've tried to illustrate what a grand bunch my colleagues were and what a grand character that Sister was and how wise. She knew that nursing was not all honey and that we had to work hard and face up to a lot of suffering and sadness and that young as we were, we just had to enjoy life as and when we could.

THE UNEXPECTED!

The cleaner at the Nurses' Home was one of the German girls who had been working on the island before the war. She was a person whom none of us could take to. She kept the place clean O.K., we had no complaint in that direction, but she certainly disliked us and her attitude said it all. Suddenly she disappeared. We thought she must have got another job somewhere else, maybe with the Germans.

The "Grape-vine" was pretty hot at this time. Things were moving fast. Germans commandeering everything they wanted and shipping many vehicles and other things over to France, no doubt to end up in Germany. Some of the German girls too were returning to their Homeland, many of them, naturally, had become very friendly with the German Officers.

We eventually heard that our cleaner had left the island. Meantime most of us found that we had lost some piece of jewellery. I was fortunate that I only lost a signet ring, but some of the Nurses had lost valuable pieces and were extremely upset. There was nothing we could do about it, the bird had flown, with our property, to the continent.

It was with mixed feelings that we heard that British submarines had been prowling up and down the Channel and that they had sunk at least one ship from here. We liked to think at the time that it was better that our property from the island was at the bottom of the sea, rather than being melted down and used in some way against the British.

As for the lives that were lost, one has just to forgive even if we cannot forget.

LIFE MUST GO ON!

I was transferred to women's surgical ward, having spent a very busy but happy time on men's surgical.

I felt very strange at first, and it seemed almost like starting again. It was quite a different atmosphere. I missed the quips and teasing from the men, but soon got into the swing of things.

Bed-pan rounds, washing backs, bed-baths, bed-making, more or less the basics, but of course different types of cases to look after.

Washing etc. seemed to take so much longer with the women patients, everything had to be just so; some could never make up their minds what to wear, pink nightie or blue nightie, particularly if it was a visiting day; and if they were lucky enough to have a choice. Not everyone had varied "wardrobes" or should I say "lockers". The hair had to be just so, irrespective of the fact it may not stay just right once on the pillow. However it was good to see them take an interest in themselves, rather than be too ill to bother. I really enjoyed the work and soon made friends with the women patients too.

It was all very interesting and such a variation of cases to learn about. Never a dull moment.

This ward had its characters too. An English lady who was a Sark resident for several years, was suffering from a fractured hip and leg and was with us for a very long time. She enjoyed helping the Nurses out and although bed-ridden and often in pain, she was frequently to be seen propped up against her pillows busy with needle and thread doing running repairs for anyone.

A lot of us did our own mending whilst on night duty. But some couldn't cope or wouldn't be bothered, so this lady was always ready to help out. I can assure you there was always plenty mending to be done.

This lady kept everyone up to date re news and all the hospital gossip. I don't mean that in a derogatory way, quite the opposite. If we wanted to check on anything, one just automatically made for the bed at the end of the ward, top corner, and nine times out of ten she'd sort things out for you. We all missed her when she was moved to a Nursing Home.

Many of the German Forces' girl friends, some locals, some French, were often admitted with various ailments, some minor and some serious. Of course there were many miscarriages included. We took it all in our stride, a patient was a patient irrespective of their background and all were treated with respect.

Some were very sad cases. We had one French girl in for an appendectomy. A lovely blond girl, very sweet. She had been brought over from Alderney (the most northerly of the C.I.'s) which had been completely evacuated. The Germans were using it as a labour camp with many foreign prisoners as slave labourers, but that is another sad story.

This French girl was a Parisian, she had been "picked up" on her way home from work one evening, I suppose you could say "kidnapped", with several other girls, and they had been brought over to Alderney for the German Officers' pleasure.

She was kept in hospital as long as possible, until the Germans became suspicious and demanded she be returned to the local prison to stay until she was fit enough to return to Alderney.

At times, when needed, I still did some voluntary St. John Ambulance duties in my hospital off-duty. That is until I had to give up St. J.A. and save all my energy for hospital work. As it happened, the day the French girl was due to leave the hospital, I was on Ambulance duty and, along with other patients ready to go home, we had quite a few calls to make in various parts of the island.

The Ambulance men were a wonderful bunch and when they realized we had the French girl on board, they delivered all the other patients home first, so that she could have a little bit longer with us. I was far from happy having to take that poor girl to the prison. The first and last time (I hope) to enter a prison. There was a bit of fuss, because we were late taking the girl in and we were made to understand how very wrong we had been. We had the feeling they would have liked to lock us up too. That girl was very grateful to us. I've often wondered what happened to her.

We frequently had Nuns as patients, which must have been quite traumatic for them, although everyone did their best to put them at their ease and respect their wishes and privacy.

Another lady we had in for a very long stay was a burns victim. She was very badly burned from the waist down and experienced so many set-backs over the eighteen months she was with us. Many times we thought we'd lose her, but no, she was a woman of great strength and courage.

It was a marvellous day when she was discharged, back on her feet again. She was an example to us all, an extremely brave lady. This patient went through a treatment for her burns that gives one the creeps to think about it. Some areas of her burns just would not heal. The poor diet did nothing to help.

She was one of the patients out on the balcony day and night. In desperation her doctor suggested that all her burns be exposed to sunlight and to leave the flies settle on the exposed flesh during the day time. Then fresh dressings be applied at night. The poor patient suffered dreadfully during the next eight hours or so as the larvae developed into maggots who worked on the wounds, eating away the "proud" flesh that surrounded the burns.

This terrible treatment did bring improvement and did help in the healing process. But the patients who received this treatment experienced such discomfort. Imagine just lying there feeling the maggots crawling over the wounds.

Dressings were a problem and scarce, especially when padding was needed, for instance, for colostomy and other leaky wounds. Where possible quantities of "tow" (coarse fibres of hemp) were used instead of cotton wool.

An appeal was made in the local 'Press' for any old linen that could be used for dressings and bandages or anything that could be of use at the hospital, but there wasn't a great response, everybody needed all the linen, or whatever, for their own use. Mothers had to make do and mend and patch over and over again. Everything was useful, even little oddments of wool which were used for darning and knitted up together for warm socks, hats etc., all colours mixed. No one minded what it looked like as long as they were warm. No mix and match in those days.

THE GERMANS INTERVENED

At the hospital things were changing too. Out of the blue the Germans decided that the Children's Home, where we Nurses were billeted, would make ideal billets for the troops. We had to be out of them within a few hours. This meant that those of us on duty had to leave the wards two by two and go up and collect our belongings and bring everything down to the hospital.

We were pretty mad about this, as we'd all settled in so well and were quite happy there. What was going to happen to us now?

As we went to collect our belongings we checked that all was well before leaving. In the cupboards were still lots of things that the children had had to leave behind. In one cupboard was a stack of small enamel chamber pots. "Look, Jerries!" exclaimed one bright spark.

Quickly all these receptacles were hauled out of the cupboard and placed in a very long line all the way down the corridor leading to the front door. We left feeling better then. I often wondered what the Germans thought of their welcome. We never heard a word from anyone about it. Hope we didn't embarrass the local representative who handed the home over.

On our arrival at the hospital we found that we had to dump our possessions in the men's side ward, which had been emptied. The patients from there had been pushed into the large ward, which made everything rather jammed up, but, hopefully, not for too long.

Several mattresses had been placed in the side ward plus bed linen, blankets and pillows and we all mucked in. Fortunately there was a toilet and bathroom off this small ward which was well used by us. The Night Staff who couldn't get home to sleep, had to bed down and try and rest during the day on the mattresses, then day staff took over the mattresses for the night. A case of turn and turn about.

Thankfully the Board of Health weren't too long getting us accommodation. They appealed to all islanders in the vicinity of the hospital, and eventually we were all found sleeping accommodation.

We missed our friends from the Home as we were all scattered amongst the community, some two at a house, some up to six, according to the rooms available. Two or three empty houses were taken over by the Board and used for Nursing Staff.

Often we would look back on our stay at the Children's Home. There was a lovely view from up there and at night time we used to watch the flares etc. over the French coast and listen to the waves of R.A.F. 'planes going over.

We later understood why we had been turned out of the Children's Home. The Germans built bunkers and gun emplacements all near the home. They too must have liked the view from up there, but, for very different reasons.

DEPORTATIONS

Orders came through that all English born residents were to report in, for deportation to Germany; men, women and children.

I helped out with one group, wearing my other hat, that of St. John Ambulance Brigade (being off from hospital that day). This particular group of deportees met at the Gaumont Cinema at the bottom of St. Julian's Avenue.

Our job was to help check that they had all necessary papers etc., answer queries, chat with them and try to cheer them up a bit. What a difficult task. Imagine how they felt, just being shipped off to the unknown, leaving everything behind them, taking only what they could carry. It was so hard to know what to say to them and many were very confused.

I was confronted with some very good friends of my parents. They were so pleased to see me before they left. It was so difficult trying to keep up a general conversation with them.

Every deportee was given a six pound size tomato chip-basket which contained food for their journey. What it consisted of I don't know, it was all well packed.

We all walked down as far as the Weighbridge, helping to carry their few bits and pieces. That's as far as we were allowed to go.

It was a sad sight to see them all go walking down the White Rock (harbour) not knowing where they were being taken.

A poignant moment for me, to have to say goodbye to a middle-aged couple I'd known all my life.

MALNUTRITION

Things didn't improve as time went by. Malnutrition and dysentery were rife. People were being admitted to the hospital for what would have normally been minor illnesses. Due to lack of the right food and comforts, plus the shortage of fuel, they were admitted and treated with whatever was available.

One of these instances which has stuck in my mind, is that of a man who was suffering from a nasty carbuncle, a family man, who died within a few days of being admitted. The poor man had no stamina left to fight off the infection which had got into his system. There were no suitable drugs available to help him fight.

Another young man, in his 20's, a haemophiliac, who had had two teeth drawn, was continually haemorrhaging. The Nurses spent night and day sitting at his bedside applying digital pressure on his gum to try and stem the flow. He must have become really fed up of having someone's fingers stuck in his mouth. He became very weak, but, thankfully we did see him return home after a very long battle.

Knowing that the Germans most probably had snake serum or some other treatment available – but not for us – made everyone more determined that we would see that young man win through.

So many patients were lost through the lack of correct medication. How many times did we hear a Doctor say, "If only we could get hold of such and such, this patient would stand a fair chance." They had the knowledge and used it to the utmost but didn't always have the "wherewithal"!

Nurses, too, had their off days and illnesses, quite a lot of dysentery and other problems, to say nothing of typhoid. Sadly we lost one well loved Nurse through typhoid and another was very ill for quite a long period, but thanks to the skill of a very dedicated person, she fully recovered.

NURSES' BILLETS

When we left the Nurses' Home, I was lucky enough to be billeted quite near the hospital, in an old cottage adjacent to a large house.

There were two nurses sharing in the next room to mine, another in a single room across the landing in the house and two Sisters in the main part, plus another nurse on the ground floor. The cottage had a small sitting area and facilities for making hot drinks.

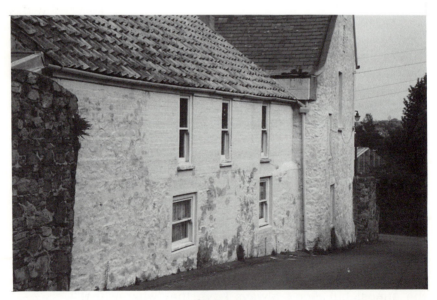

Cottage

Our landlord and his wife were very pleasant people and always ready for a chat when we came and went to and from the hospital. They must have found it very strange having so many using their home. We were all careful not to intrude on their privacy. We respected their home and kept to our rooms.

The landlady kept our rooms clean. One would hear her banging around with the hoover, singing hymns, which was not a very welcome sound when one was trying to sleep after a hard night's work.

It was understood that we were not allowed to entertain anyone in our rooms – But, of course, "rules are made to be broken".

I heard of the following little episode one morning when I had just come off night duty. The landlady informed me there had been fun and games the previous evening.

Apparently the two Nurses in the next room to mine had smuggled in a local lad to spend the evening with them, until he had to return before curfew. However, the landlord had a feeling that something was going on, and went up to check. He asked the girls if everything was alright.

"Oh, yes thanks," they assured him. The landlord stayed chatting to them for a while when suddenly the wardrobe moved and fell face down. The landlord went to lift it back.

"We'll do that Mr. ... We can manage, please don't worry."

But the game was up. A very embarrassed young man clambered out, thankfully none the worse for his fall and no damage was done to the wardrobe. We all had a good laugh. But the householders felt they were responsible for us and didn't want any "carryings on" in their home, which was understandable.

The landlord had deliberately kept the girls chatting, because he had seen the lad's bike at the back of the cottage.

He was just waiting for something to happen. Looking back, he certainly handled things very well, it can't have been easy having us all under his roof, particularly as they were a middle-aged couple, with no family of their own.

At the top of the cottage stairs, was what was called the bathroom for the use of everyone in the house and the cottage.

We, of the Nursing Staff, were very fortunate that we could use the staff bathrooms at the hospital, which was a good thing because the "bathroom" at the "digs" consisted of a wash-stand with a china bowl and jug of cold water, with a bucket under the stand to empty used water into. There was just about enough room to stand and wash. No indoors W.C., one had to walk up the garden, behind some outbuildings to use the toilet.

If one used the bowl and jug, to maybe wash hands and face and brush teeth – having emptied the water into the bucket, one felt the least one could do was to trudge up the garden to empty it, which was rather a bind and it was very awkward during curfew, as we had no choice but to use chamber pots, then come morning it was another walk up the garden to empty that bucket again!

During one spell of night duty, I went to bed first thing that morning as I'd arranged an outing for late afternoon and was on duty again that night.

I enjoyed a good sleep in, then was awakened by the trusty alarm. Remembering I had a date, I jumped out of bed thinking a good splash in cold water would really wake me up and bring me to my senses pretty quickly. I dashed to the "bathroom". (Here I must explain the "bathroom" door opened outwards.) I flung the "bathroom" door open only to find our landlord sitting in a tin washing tray with his knees up to his chin having a bath. I closed the door quickly feeling a bit of a fool. He was very short-sighted and had muttered something about being ready to have his back washed. I assumed he must have thought it was his wife who opened the door. I just didn't wait to see or explain anything.

So much for a refreshing wash that day.

I never knew if he found out who it was that disturbed him, I didn't enquire.

There were two other Nurses in the house across the road. Their landlord was rather an odd character. He was a grower prior to the occupation and always seemed to be very busy around his property, which was quite near the hospital grounds. He was the sort of chap who just had to know everything that was going on. He'd spend quite a lot of his time in the hospital gardens chatting to the gardeners or anyone else he could find at the time.

We got quite used to him appearing suddenly over a hedge, or walking innocently behind us as we made our way back to our "digs". It wasn't a very nice feeling when it was dusk and some of the girls were a bit frightened of him.

Getting a bit fed up with him, the next time we sensed he was there listening to us, I said: "Good-night Mr. .... ". There was a lot of scrambling about and we knew for sure that it was him. He never approached any of us and was really quite harmless, just gave us the 'creeps'.

One funny thing about him was his trilby hat, which he always wore. From the brim of the hat he had a piece of string hanging downwards and attached to the stem of his pipe. We could never quite work out if the string was anchoring his hat to his head via the pipe, or if having few teeth, the string was helping to hold his pipe in his mouth.

The German troops were well spread out all over the island. There were several near our cottage as they now had gun emplacements at the top of the hill. Many Germans were living in houses of their choice, having turned out the occupants at short notice.

This was cunning, as having troops integrated with the islanders, it lowered the risk of having the R.A.F. paying a visit. This way the Germans were safe. But <u>so were we</u>.

The Germans were extremely nervous and jumpy. We had many a laugh at their expense. As soon as they heard a 'plane, they'd run like mad and fire at anything anywhere. They were kept quite busy because the R.A.F. frequently flew over the islands on their way to the continent.

As much as we hated being occupied, we must admit that on the whole the forces were very well behaved.

The Nursing Staff carried night passes, as shifts often necessitated us going back and forth during curfew hours. I can honestly say we weren't nervous at being out on the road at those times and, to my knowledge, no Nurse was ever accosted or troubled by a German. Maybe it was the uniform they respected. On looking back I realize, we just felt safe.

CYCLES EVERYWHERE

There were many strange sights on the roads. Cycles and shanks' pony were the main way of getting about. Cycles of all shapes and sizes were in continual use, many of the models being made up of various bits and pieces. Old bikes that had been left lying about for years because they weren't needed any more, were now very precious and a popular mode of transport.

A little cobbler who lived nearby was very resourceful and helped out many islanders, not only with shoe repairing. His customers had to supply the necessary material for their repairs be it odd bits of leather or rubber, but he always managed to do a good job. He was also good at repairing cycle tyres. He'd manage to stitch patches on to the worn parts of the tyre. It made the ride a bit bumpy, but was more comfortable than the hose-pipe tyre which many people were using. There'd be an almighty 'bump' every time the join in the hose-pipe tyre hit the road.

Another useful "gadget" was the cycle trailer, an ideal contrivance for carting various items from A to B. It consisted of a box on two wheels; old pram ones were ideal if they could be found. A bar was attached to the base or axle of the cart, which extended up and over the cycle's back wheel, then bolted on to the cycle frame just below the saddle.

Clothing was becoming very worn and patched and many men wore socks that were more darns than the original socks or had multi-coloured ones in stripes of all colours which had been knitted up. Old worn garments were ripped and the best parts of the wool salvaged to make up hats, scarves and mitts. We all wore wool pixie hoods that were just the thing to keep one warm when cycling.

One morning in town I bumped into my landlady and was amazed to see she was wearing one of my pixie hoods. Yes, I was lucky – I possessed two. She was very embarrassed, poor woman, and didn't know what to say. It must have been when she was cleaning my room that she saw it and thought she'd borrow it as it was a very cold day.

Eventually, she stammered out her apologies and said she thought I wouldn't mind her using it. Of course I didn't really mind, but it would have been nice to have been asked. As I was on nights at the time I told her to let me have any bits of double knitting wool she had and that I'd knit one for her when I had a chance.

She duly passed on the wool one night as I was going on duty. Imagine her surprise when I presented her with her very own hood the next morning. We had had a slack night and I had managed to make her hood. I can still see her to this day proudly wearing her knitted hat. I don't think she went out without it until after Liberation. It was almost as colourful as Joseph's coat, with its variety of stripes. No one was fashion conscious in those days, but only too pleased to keep ourselves warm.

We had our share of Births, Marriages and Deaths among the relatives of the Staff. Everyone seemed to know everyone else's business and felt as if we were one big family, who shared each other's joys and sorrows.

One marriage that stands out in the memory was between a Nurse and a St. John Ambulance Officer. The wedding ceremony was at the Câtel Church and many of the "off duty" Staff went up to see our colleague "off". The couple came out of Church to find a Guard of Honour of Nursing and the St. John Ambulance Staff. Two stretchers and bearers awaited the Happy Couple. With much laughter and ribbing they were carried down the long pathway to the gate where the horse and carriage stood ready waiting to carry them off. There were other Staff weddings at various times but they were more traditional.

HOSPITAL "WAY OF LIFE"

Because of the rationing, when we visited friends or relatives we always took what we could in the way of food.

I remember walking out to St. Peter's with a friend to visit some relatives one Sunday afternoon. We had managed to save some bits and pieces and made up a pudding of sorts with milk. It had turned out something like a bread pudding. We carried it all the way out there, very pleased with our contribution.

One of the ways to warm food was to place it in a covered dish under the fire basket in the grate, where it would heat through. This particular day we must have left it too long and our wonderful "pudding" was burnt. Still we all enjoyed it just the same. We were very hungry after our long walk.

— — — —

One always seemed to meet ex patients in the town, besides other friends and relatives. One day I was stopped by a woman who said, "Hello Nurse, I've been wanting to see you."

"Oh yes, Mrs. ..., how are you and how is your daughter getting on?"

"That's what I want to talk to you about. I just can't get her to settle down at night. What did you do to help her sleep?"

"I'm sorry, but I don't think I did anything special for her."

"But you must have done. She always says I don't make her pillows comfy like Nurse ... did. Now what's the secret?"

That poor mother must have felt so inadequate. I really think that "Young Madam" must have been playing up. However after a nice chat with Mum and an explanation as to how I arranged the pillows, I sincerely hope things improved.

As I have said, we were such a close community during those years, everyone knew each other. At times one would have to look twice when greeted with a "Hello Nurse", as people dressed and walking about can look so different from a very ill person lying in bed.

We met such a variety of characters in the hospital, both patients, Nursing, and Domestic Staff.

I was happy working on Male Surgical where I first began to learn the hospital way of life. The Nursing Staff on at that time were a good crowd to work with and I was proud to be one of their number.

The Irish Sister who was in charge of that ward at the time soon discovered that she had a very inquisitive probationer on her hands, and I must say she was very good to me. Once she realized how interested I was, she took a lot of trouble in showing me many things. We had no formal training, we were taught the practicalities and did our own swotting when we could get hold of the relevant books.

Sister would call me over to watch the different types of dressings and treatments, and made me scrub up and help at times, which was in my opinion the best way to learn. I was very grateful to her, nothing was too much trouble, she was easy to approach if ever I had any queries, as were most of the senior staff.

One morning I was summoned to a patient's bedside. "Now Nurse, Mr. ... is prepared for theatre and ready for his pre-med. injection. It's here ready on the tray for you." I just looked at her. "Come along now, they'll be fetching him in soon."

I was petrified. Poor man, I thought, little does he know that I have never given an injection in my life (there was no practising on oranges in those days). Trying to look more confident than I felt, I swabbed his arm, picked up the syringe, cleared the air bubble, then placed the needle at the correct angle, as I had seen many times, trying to remember all I'd been told. As I hesitated, the needle just flew in. Sister had been standing by watching and had nudged my elbow just at the right time. That was the first of many injections that I was to give. I never minded giving them to adults, but always felt very mean when having to inject a child.

Out on the veranda there were approximately five beds, three of which were occupied by long stay patients who were T.B. cases. They were a cheerful bunch and always ready with a "quip" at the Nurses, causing many a laugh. As they were overlooking the yard, they saw all the comings of Ambulances, Doctors' cars and later the Doctors' cycles.

There was also the outdoor staff, farmworkers, gardeners, and many of the Nursing Staff coming and going on and off duty, because the cycle stands were beneath the verandas. They so enjoyed a chat with anyone passing by, who would spend a bit of time with them. Sad to say in those days there was no real cure for T.B.

The other end of the veranda was used by various patients at different times. Some just enjoyed being outdoors. There were canvas curtains which helped keep out the worst of the weather, that, plus hot water bottles and loads of blankets, kept them all cosy and happy.

Before we had a Children's Ward, the children were in with the adults. One young boy suffering from burns was out on the balcony and the men helped keep him happy and continually encouraged him. His burns were very stubborn at healing. Doctors tried everything they could, until eventually with the co-operation of the parents, it was decided to try a skin graft, taking the skin from the child's father. There was no way of testing to see if the skin was suitable or not, but it was worth a try.

I'm happy to say it was some success. The surgeon had never done a skin graft before, all this was explained to the parents prior to the operation. The boy was discharged later when it was seen that a good job had been accomplished.

That boy has become a well respected islander. I don't know how much of his ordeal he remembers, he was only four years old at the time, a very brave little boy, loved by patients and staff.

It was quite an experience learning the hospital way of life. There were so many new faces and so many different characters.

The Domestic Staff too had quite an influence on us, in their own way. Nurses were not always popular with them. If things were left in a mess or we either forgot or didn't have time to do what we should, "Those Nurses" weren't allowed to forget it. Still, they were very good workers and always willing to help out when and where they could in spite of the moans.

They often helped to serve patients' meals and clear up trays from the ward and did all the dishes, besides the cleaning. One elderly lady in particular had a very long face, it was hard work to get her to smile, and no one could hurry her. She was a very hard worker and certainly took great pride in her work, everything was spotless.

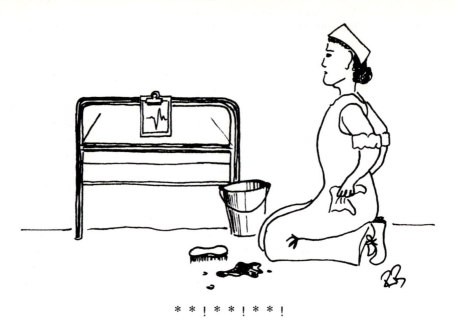

* * ! * * ! * * !

Then there was Lizzie who worked with her. Lizzie did all the rough work, all the dirtiest jobs, she was <u>always</u> full of chat. The male patients were greatly amused by her dry way of talking. Whenever she became annoyed her language was rather colourful. She didn't care what anyone thought. When scrubbing the ward floor it was done with much vigour, plus quite a lot of noise, clanking the galvanized bucket on the floor.

As I have mentioned before, the ward had to be spick and span before Matron came to do her morning round, which was more of an inspection than anything else.

One particular morning Lizzie had not finished her floor when Matron walked in and, as there was one critically ill patient in the ward, Matron asked her if she could be a bit quieter as she was disturbing the patient making such a noise with her bucket.

Much to our amazement, Lizzie just sat back on her heels, looked up at Matron and said: "If you don't want me to make so much noise, you'd better get somebody to fix some bl....... rubber handles on the ...... buckets"! and promptly continued with her scrubbing.

A deadly silence descended on the ward, no one, patients or staff, knew <u>what</u> to say. Matron on her dignity just turned and walked out of the ward. Then we all collapsed in laughter. Knowing what I know now, I bet that's just what Matron was doing too. She had a great personality and though she could put the fear of God into anyone, be it Doctor, Nursing Staff or patient, she had a wonderful sense of humour and a heart of gold.

There was one young man who had got into trouble with the Germans — I can't recall for what. He had escaped from a small group as they were being marched down St. Julian's Avenue to the boat, escorted by German Guards. This lad had suddenly stopped, bent down to do up his shoe lace and the next minute had sprinted through the side streets. He was a fit sports-loving person and had made a very quick get away. He was at large for several days, no one knew where he was.

Going off duty one evening a colleague and I were confronted with Ambulance men bearing a stretcher, we stood aside for them to enter the ward, the Nurse beside me gasped and under her breath said; "I'm sure that's .... on that stretcher, I'm going back to find out." The missing lad was a relation of hers and as there was a police escort with the party, I guessed she was right.

Unfortunately for him, whilst on the run, he chose to climb over a wall which had pieces of glass inserted on the top, and he cut both his hands very badly. He had made his way to a Doctor's Surgery, but there was no way he could be attended to there, he had to be admitted, in any case it was too big a risk for anyone to take, so he agreed to give himself up to the local police and he was attended to straightway. Everything was reported to the Germans and the local police had the job of guarding him night and day in the hospital where he was kept as long as possible until he was well enough to be deported.

"INCIDENTS!"

In the early days many people were very nervous of the Germans and there were many silly accidents. One never knew when or where a German would appear. While doing an ordinary everyday job of work some of them would delight in making a local nervous.

This happened to one chap while he was loading heavy boxes on the back of a lorry. He was bending down arranging these heavy items when, out of the corner of his eye, he saw a German lingering around watching. Being a nervous sort of fellow he continued what he was doing, but, with one eye on the soldier and not paying enough attention to what he was doing. Unfortunately, he jammed himself between the heavy boxes and he was trapped in a very painful area. I'm afraid I don't remember what treatment he received in hospital, but once he was well again he received a lot of teasing from his mates. It took a long time for him to live down that little accident.

There were many road accidents due to having to ride on the right-hand side of the road.

One young man was out delivering milk. This was at the beginning of the occupation, before islanders had to collect everything from depots. The young chap was knocked over by a German vehicle and was brought into hospital deeply unconscious, in quite a bad way. I can't remember if there were any other injuries, I think it was just the fractured skull. He was unconscious for a very long time and we were very concerned.

Then one Sunday evening – we still had a radio in the ward at the time – the hymn singing was on and some of the men joined in, when suddenly we were all very surprised to hear a very strong voice coming from behind the screens, joining in with "Onward Christians Soldiers." From that time on he never looked back, he made an excellent recovery and, much to everyone's delight, was soon back on his feet again.

Men's surgical ward always seemed to be busy. Having hospital treatment until things settled down a bit was quite frequently used by both males and females. The Doctors became wise to it all and the Germans were tricked more than once. Thank goodness the Germans never "cottoned on". Those Doctors are un-sung heroes.

We had some Police Officers in with various minor troubles which needed surgery and a few days in hospital, i.e. hernia, appendix, etc. They had "acquired" a few bits and pieces from the German stores and used their stay in hospital as a sanctuary until the heat died down a bit. Some did serve time in the local prison for their misdeeds and were extremely lucky not to be deported. Those on the ward at least shared the fruits of their labours with other patients. The men were only too pleased to have a few treats to liven up "the 'orrible 'ospital grub!" In truth, for some, the hospital "grub" was a bit better than they would have had at home.

A local man was brought in by the German authorities for treatment. He was under punishment, for what, we never knew. He had been kept at work, in the dark, underground, attending some boilers for the forces. Kept in the boiler room night and day, he was brought in for treatment on his eyes.

The hospital management had received strict instructions that he was to receive only the bare necessities and kept on his own as a prisoner. They agreed for him to be placed in a "padded cell" which was just off the ward. It's not as bad as it sounds, quite a nice little room, a window with bars and a pleasant outlook over fields.

As soon as the men on the ward heard what was happening, they insisted on sending down a few bits and pieces that they could spare, plus reading matter and flowers.

On duty one afternoon with my friend (Laurel & Hardy together again), we had to bed-bath this prisoner. Having done our duty we left him fresh and clean with the paper and a lovely vase of flowers, which helped to cheer him up in his cell, and made our way back to the main ward, when, who should we see but Matron slowly escorting a huge German Officer up the ward towards us.

We just turned back, carefully closing all the doors behind us. The poor man in the cell must have thought we'd gone mad as we cleared all the "extras" that he wasn't allowed and darted into the bathroom adjacent until Matron and the Officer were in the cell, when we rushed back to the main ward to continue our duties there, trying not to look too scared or guilty.

We were very busy when they came back from the cell and it was with great trepidation that I went to open the ward door for Matron and the Officer.

The patient was so grateful to us when we went back to check how he was. He was soon well enough to return to his work. It was quite some time later we heard that he had passed away, how or why I do not recall. I don't think we ever heard exactly what had happened to him.

The men on the wards certainly made the best of things and those who smoked were always very busy. You can't imagine what they smoked and you wouldn't believe the aroma that wafted across the ward. Let's face it, due to the diet we were quite used to a variety of smells and the "whiffs" from the smokers did nothing to help. One chap would be rubbing up dried rose petals, another cutting up dried leaves and stalks with scissors, anything that could burn would be tried out.

Growing tobacco plants was quite popular, the leaves would be dried, some prepared with secret ingredients and those who could afford Black Market prices would add some spirit such as rum to add to the flavour and smell of the tobacco. The leaves having been impregnated with a little spirit were pressed into cakes, then sliced and rubbed up. This would all take a great deal of time, trial and error. The various concoctions would keep the pipes going and the cigarette smokers would roll their own.

When cigarette papers ran out they'd use tissue or any other thin paper. Some patients couldn't or just wouldn't do without their smoke, much to the disgust of everyone else. At times the ward smelt just like a bonfire.

Talking of paper reminds me that in time the hospital ran out of toilet paper, or, toilet rolls to be precise. Thanks to someone's brilliant thinking we had supplies of paper the type of which had been used by growers for lining tomato trays and baskets. It was an assortment of colours, blue, green, red and yellow. The colours had been a way of grading the tomatoes. The paper was cut up into suitable size, the squares then banded into packets and sold for everyone's use, though many folk resorted to the use of printed paper and even books for this purpose. At least the packing paper put a bit of colour into our lives.

Many men had employment with the Germans – they had no choice, it was that or nothing. Some of the more alert men enjoyed taking risks and what they could sabotage they would. Better still if they could smuggle <u>out</u> some things <u>for</u> the missus and the kids, they did! Who could blame them?

Farmers were badly hampered by curfew and had little enough to feed their cattle. They would leave the cattle out to grass overnight, only to find the next morning that an animal was missing, or some of the cows had been milked.

One farmer who we had as a patient, happened to be out after curfew tending a sick cow, when he was shot in the leg by an over enthusiastic sentry. The farmer was laid up for a long while and was very lucky to get back on his feet again.

Another farmer-grower I knew who often found his cows had been milked overnight, was determined to do something about it. His two sons took up the challenge. The cows were staked out for the night near the greenhouses, a short distance from the house. The two sons, taking a risk, settled down for the night in deck chairs inside the greenhouse, where they could see the cows. Being out there was against all rules and regulations, as it was after curfew.

Sure enough, in the middle of the night came two Germans. When they were well settled down to milking, they were very rudely interrupted, one ran for his life, the other was not quite so lucky. These two soldiers were known to the brothers and had often passed the time of day with them. The next day the soldiers sheepishly bade the family, "Good morning," as usual and when one was asked what had happened to him, very ashamed but with a grin, said: "Black-eye; milking cows last night".

Those cows were safe after that episode. But, I suppose some other poor farmer suffered.

Fortunately those Germans my friends had encountered were understanding and thank goodness, not armed, or there could have been very serious consequences.

NIGHT DUTY

My first night-duty was on the men's ward. I enjoyed night work very much.

Again it was a case of learning a different routine, but I coped O.K. and I already knew several of the patients, having been on "days" with them, and they were a great help, always ready to put "Nurse" right.

I soon got into the swing of things, learning to sleep in the day-time, which was a bit difficult at first, but after a few hectic nights I didn't need any "rocking to sleep".

A few nights on and one of the men passed away. He was quite an elderly gentleman and ironically I had known him all my life. He was an old neighbour, but that's neither here nor there.

The senior Nurse to me was a bit of a "Madam". I had worked with her many times before on days. A junior could never do anything right for her, and here was I having the honour of helping her to lay out the old chap.

We had been rushed off our feet for most of the night and were very tired, and had to hurry with this job to finish before we had to wake the ward for 5 a.m. washings.

We were coping very well between us when suddenly my senior said "Come on Nurse, hurry up, take this bandage and tie his feet together, you do know how to do that I hope?" Feeling very tired, I got the giggles and didn't know how to keep a straight face. "But Nurse", I began. "What now, haven't you done that simple job yet?" "Sorry Nurse, but no,. I can't." "And why not, have I got to do everything myself? And stop your giggling." – Oh Dear – "I'm sorry Nurse, but this man has had his leg amputated; I can't tie his feet together as he only has one foot!"

This was all conducted in whispers so as not to disturb other patients. It took a long time for that little episode to be forgotten. Once again my sense of humour almost got me into "dead" trouble.

During slack nights, we'd all enjoy a sit down and a gossip. On the men's ward we were usually a Senior Nurse, one Junior and one Male Nurse. Night Sister would overlook the male and female wards.

We'd have our main meal at mid-night, two shifts, with female surgical staff. At 4 a.m. it was tea-time, which we each took in our own ward's kitchen.

As I was saying it was great to sit and chat or read and maybe knit. We would take it in turns to do the rounds, checking that everyone was alright.

One male nurse used to amuse us. He always volunteered to do the rounds for us. We suddenly realized why. The poor chap suffered a great deal with flatulence, so, he'd trot down the ward very efficiently with a cacophony of sound echoing through the ward. Needless to say we had great difficulty keeping straight and innocent faces as he came back to report that all was well, assuming that we'd think the patients were responsible for all the noises.

On another night duty stint, we had a patient who <u>never slept</u>. This man was in with a fractured femur and not a very happy man. He was never grateful for anything that was done for him, he just moaned and complained about everything and everybody. There was no pleasing him at all.

Every morning he complained to his Doctor that he hadn't slept all night, it was either noisy, or the Nurses didn't make him comfortable, and he had such a lot of pain. This was in spite of having had pain killers.

The Day Sister assured the Doctor that his patient was reported as having had a good night. Still the man complained.

Finally the Night Sister had just about had enough of his nonsense. We nurses on duty with her at that time were ordered around this man's bed, and Sister told us to be sure to watch what was about to happen; this was approximately 1.20 a.m. We'd just finished dinner. The patient concerned was sound asleep. The Sister opened his locker, removed his pipe and tobacco (such as it was), filled the pipe and then placed the pipe stem in his mouth which was wide open.

Of course he awoke with a start and, in language I could not repeat here, demanded to know what on earth was happening and what was the idea of bl..... well waking him up in the middle of the night. Night Sister, very sweet and apologetic, said how very sorry she was to have disturbed him, but, as it had been reported so many times that he hadn't slept a wink since being admitted, she really thought he would enjoy having a smoke to pass the time away. By this time the whole ward was awake, enjoying every bit of the goings on.

They were fed up with the cantankerous old boy's behaviour, and it took a bit of time getting them all settled down once more.

As you will have guessed, there was never another sleepless night complaint from that quarter. He continued having "good" nights throughout his stay.

THROWN IN AT THE DEEP END!

The Night Sister was the one who was always surprising me by making me do things I hadn't done before.

We had an emergency case in one night, a man with a strangulated hernia.

Having admitted him and made him as comfortable as possible, I was approached by Sister. "Now Nurse, along with you to theatre!" "Me, Sister?" "Yes, Nurse, you, now go and get scrubbed up!" "But I've never done any theatre work." "That's alright, now don't worry, Theatre Nurse will tell you what to do, just shadow her and help her when she needs help".

Gosh! Talk about being thrown in at the deep end, especially in the middle of the night. I had no fear of what I was about to witness. I only hoped I wouldn't make a fool of myself by touching something or doing anything I shouldn't.

"Hurry Nurse, we'll be bringing in the patient very shortly!"

I enjoyed every minute of that operation and was most intrigued by the skill of the surgeon. He always welcomed Nurses and would take a lot of trouble explaining what he was doing and why.

That was my first theatre duty. I came out of there on cloud nine and starving, thankfully the others had kept my meal hot. I just sat and tucked in, thinking how lucky I was to be in such an interesting and exciting job.

With continued changing circumstances, night duty was made more difficult with very limited lighting on the wards. Oil filled small empty lemonade crystal bottles, with a piece of shoe lace inserted through the lid to act as a wick, was tried out as night-lights, but these caused a very smoky and smelly atmosphere, not good for anyone's chest.

At times a Staff Nurse would stand in for Night Sister and this little episode concerns such an occasion.

We were receiving some goods from France at this time, many of which were a bit strange to us. Toiletries such as tooth paste and soap came in blocks of similar size, both very "gritty" but better than nothing. The soap rations we had received before, locally produced, had a very unpleasant smell, so the French soap was an improvement. There was a very respected local man who used to travel to France, with German permission, to purchase what he could for the islanders. He was very brave to face these journeys and approach the French, who must have had little to spare. We owe a lot to our fellow islander who took such risks.

However, I'm straying from the point. At times washing a patient at 5 a.m. in half light was no joke. More than once I found I was using tooth paste instead of soap and wondered why the patient looked so pale.

This particular night had been hectic, as we had another death in the ward. The Acting Sister very kindly volunteered to lay out this patient as she knew we had a lot of heavy cases to deal with that morning, all the washes and everything else that went with the morning rush.

Dashing around from bed to bed in the half light with washing bowls of water, I realized that Staff Nurse, who was supposedly laying out the patient, was sitting in the duty room doubled up as if in pain. When I got there to check what was wrong, I saw she was crying with laughter, not a bit like the very efficient Staff Nurse we all knew and respected. It took a bit of time to get any sense as to what was making her laugh so much.

She had been washing the deceased and found that the soap just wouldn't lather, so in her frustration had gone into the duty room where the large windows let in more light. There, she discovered that she had been using a piece of <u>hard cheese</u>.

Everyone had received a small ration that day. Staff Nurse had felt around in the locker and found what she thought was a small block of soap, in poor light she had been unable to identify what it was.

After a spell of night duty it was so good to have a few days off before going back on days. It was a great opportunity to catch up on the way the rest of the island was doing.

I was fortunate in having relatives and friends to visit. Some would insist on sharing a meal, but as I could have regular meals at the hospital, such as they were, I didn't impose unless I was sure they had sufficient to share.

My father was living alone, but my married sister and relatives saw to it that he was alright. Much against his principles he was working as a driver for the Germans, there was no choice. He had to drive the Officers around the island on various inspections of the troops, etc. He was not very happy, but those he was working for were quite pleasant. It meant a lot of waiting about and working all hours, but at least he occasionally got a meal out of them.

I tried to visit my grandparents pretty regularly. My grandfather had been a grower-farmer and tried to keep some of the growing side going. The Germans always claimed a percentage of all crops grown.

One morning, whilst at my grandparents, I took a walk over the fields, it was quite early. I found several leaflets scattered about which the R.A.F. had dropped during the night. We received these every so often. Some were printed in English, which would give us a few facts, and some were printed in German, these of course they considered as being propaganda. We were glad to know we were not forgotten and enjoyed reading and catching up with a bit of world news, not a lot, but it helped.

While picking up a few leaflets I glanced down the valley to see there was a group of soldiers with shovels and a lorry and a very irate German Officer shouting at the men to hurry. Apparently the bulk of the leaflets had dropped down there, they hadn't scattered very far. Realizing I should be in trouble if seen, I hid a few leaflets about me and made my way back to the house. It was absolutely "*verboten*"! to pick any leaflet up. I don't remember what those leaflets contained that day, but was taking no chances. I hid a couple in the pig-sty (no pigs in these at the time). If any search was to be carried out I wanted to be sure there weren't any to be found in the house.

I then decided to cycle to my father's, to let him have a copy or two. However, once again, I had to be careful as I had to pass along the road where the Germans were building their underground hospital. When we saw all the work going on there, once again rumour was rife. There was talk of the Gas Chambers. Knowing even the troops were getting short of food, were they that desperate? Did they intend reducing the population? What thoughts went through our heads. Who could blame us? Thank God it was all unfounded, and we were later to see wounded soldiers sitting on top of the hillock enjoying a bit of fresh air.

Having stuck a couple of leaflets in my shoes and a couple up in the handle-bars of the bike, I hoped for the best. Thankfully everything went well.

On passing the underground hospital it was a pitiful sight to see so many foreign labourers working so hard and the guards standing over them with fixed bayonets. One daren't look too interested, I just had to pedal on my way, as if nothing was happening.

Later, when the underground hospital was finished, many wounded were brought over from France and on a sunny day one would often see soldiers on crutches, some with arms in slings, others with head bandaged, sitting on the hillside on the top of their hospital, enjoying a bit of fresh air.

FORCED LABOURERS

The labour forces were used to build bunkers, gun emplacements and other defences. They were men from many different countries; French, Spaniards, Japanese, African, Chinese, Poles, Rumanians, etc. They all looked so sorrowful, half starved, without suitable clothing, being pushed and shoved around. Some could hardly stand but were still made to work until they dropped and had to be carried back to their camp by fellow prisoners.

The only clothing these men had was what they were wearing at the time of their capture, no change or replacements. What a sorry sight they were when marched to work every morning; clothes in rags, a lot of them with no shoes as such, just bits of rag and the remains of footwear tied together as best they could, looking so dejected and so ill.

Meeting a group on their way to slave labour made one feel so inadequate. While the German soldiers just hustled and hurried them along, one just had to stand aside while they all filed past.

And we felt sorry for ourselves! No one dared help these poor men, they were very closely guarded as they went along the road.

An uncle of mine, a grower whose property bordered one of the camps, felt so sorry for them that he risked being caught by placing vegetables that he could spare on the hedge which divided the properties. He hid root vegetables under the weeds and hedge-cuttings. The men knew where to look and were extremely grateful, but, they too had to be careful and make sure they were not seen gathering the vegetables which they often ate raw. I hate to think of the consequences should my uncle or any of those men have been found out.

Many of the men in forced labour lost their lives and were buried in a field near Les Vauxbelets. At the end of hostilities all the remains were exhumed and given a proper burial.

Anything in the way of the 'Jack Boot' was blown up and demolished, be it a home or any other building. So much agricultural land too was spoilt forever to make way for their concrete monstrosities.

RADIOS CONFISCATED

Many islanders had hidden radios, and cats' whiskers, which was strictly *"verboten"*. They had all supposedly been "handed in" along with all cameras and fire arms.

The instructions for building "cats' whiskers" had been on leaflets which had been dropped by the R.A.F. These little radios were ideal for hiding and people who didn't have any head-phones found telephone receivers were very useful. Many sets were hidden in very unusual places in the home, outhouses, sheds, amongst junk. I even heard of one being kept in a saucepan on the hearth. One never knew when the Germans might decide to make a search, maybe having been "tipped off" by some so-called "friend" or other.

At the time of the Duke of Kent's funeral, I can well remember sitting in a friend's house at the piano, not that I could play, no, I was there for a very different reason. The piano was near the window which looked out on to the back door. I was sitting there listening in to the funeral service of H.R.H. Duke of Kent, with head-phones on and yes, you've guessed it, bang in the middle of the service, a German Officer appeared at the door. Oh dear! Panic stations!

I dared not move too quickly in case I attracted his attention. I was thankful that he had his back to me and hoped and prayed that I could move everything quietly and be able to act normally. I managed to remove the head-phones and place them back in the music seat without being seen and with my back to the window pretended to be very busy sorting out music sheets. It all took just a matter of seconds but to my friends and me it seemed like hours.

I can't remember what the Officer was there for, but we were all very relieved when he went on his way, he hadn't even stepped in the doorway. I was terrified by the thought that through me my friends could have been in very serious trouble. I just don't know what would have happened, probably a spell in prison in France, as an example to others who may be hiding radios.

The set was transferred to another hiding place after that little episode. I don't know where and didn't want to know. Suffice to say that I knew that any news I heard in that household was genuine, not rumour.

I did so appreciate those good friends. I was always made most welcome and passed many happy "off duty" times with the whole family.

They were very good folk and helped many of their less fortunate neighbours, who were having difficulty keeping body and soul together. Many times I accompanied the daughter of the house for walks through the lanes, visiting elderly folk who lived on their own. There was always a little basket of goodies handed over. Little extras that cheered the elderly people.

The majority of the islanders were like one big happy family, always ready to help each other. I say majority because, as always happens at times like these, there are those who forget the meaning of loyalty to say nothing of dignity.

ENTERTAINMENT

It was good to get away from the hospital atmosphere now and then. We were allowed to visit the cinema (Gaumont) to view German films with English sub-titles, plus news reels filled with propaganda.

I went once, more out of curiosity than anything else. The forces were sitting on one side of the cinema and the civilians on the other side. It seemed to me that there was an uncomfortable feeling – I didn't like the atmosphere one bit, sitting there with German troops too close for comfort, even though there was a rope rail down the middle of the centre aisle. The Nurse I was with at the time was somewhat of a giggler and kept nudging me during the News Reels. I was terrified that we would get told off and possibly be shown out, or something equally drastic. We of course did see the funny side of things. According to the German News, England was well and truly finished or should I say "*Kaput*". The North Cinema on the Bridge, St. Sampson's was also used by islanders and troops. Quite a few locals regularly visited the cinemas – more for something to do I should imagine.

The local Amateur Dramatic Society put on many plays and variety shows at the Little Theatre, and very good they were too. It was a great way to relax and forget all the troubles for a couple of hours, even though there'd be a few of those hated uniforms in the audience with their girl friends. Naturally our local comedians had to watch their "patter" when we were graced with the presence of the forces.

Another thing enjoyed by many were the private dances (by invitation only) at Sunnycroft Hotel. Anyone could hire the ballroom for an evening's dancing, with a three piece band providing the music. We spent many a happy time there, meeting up with friends and there was no chance of unwanted 'guests' turning up.

Sometimes it was a rush to get back home before curfew, but the old bikes stood up to a lot of rough treatment and it was a race to see who could get down the Rohais fastest and back to the hospital first.

Winter curfew was at 9 p.m., 10 p.m. in the summer. We changed the clocks one hour as British time, then a month later another hour as continental time.

Everyone enjoyed the long summer evenings to the best of their ability.

Most beaches and surrounding areas were mined, but we did have some areas which were safe for swimming.

During the winter months the family gatherings were generally all-night affairs; everyone took their rations with them and made their own entertainment one way or another.

VISITING TIMES

Life at the hospital continued much the same. Spells of night duty, day duty and theatre work. Patients came and patients went, never a dull moment. Always busy, not only on the surgical wards where I was working, but also on the medical wards and, of course, the maternity ward too was always busy.

As nursing staff from all wards always met up in the dining and recreation rooms, you can imagine we swopped many an interesting and at times very amusing story.

Visiting days were the highlight of the patients' stay. Two nurses received visitors at the top of the stairs to direct them into the right ward.

There was never a lot that relatives could bring their loved ones, whatever was brought in was probably a little tit-bit that one of the family had given up from their own meagre rations.

If, however, it was someone who could afford Black Market prices, then there would be treats, even one teaspoonful of real tea, not the bramble leaf one that everyone was used to. If a patient was fortunate enough to receive a little real tea, then, that small amount was stewed and stewed again on top of the duty room Aga. It was amazing the number of patients (and nurses) who were cheered up by a lovely refreshing "cuppa", the flavour was out of this world, stewed or not.

Another thing that cheered everyone was the flowers. That was one thing the Germans couldn't erase from our island. We received many beautiful blooms on the wards. But, some flowers were "taboo". Never did we arrange red flowers with white blooms together in one vase, that was very unlucky. All was well if you remembered to put a different coloured bloom amongst them, better still, if possible, was a fine arrangement of RED, WHITE AND BLUE flowers. Most patriotic!

Should anyone dare to bring in "arum lilies", well, that was a sure sign of death. So, after a hasty explanation to the recipient, the lilies were spirited away to the mortuary. Most patients were only too happy to see the back of them.

Many of the visitors looked as bad, if not worse, than the patients. Having to walk back and forth, sometimes from quite a distance, often feeling weak and tired, they were only too thankful to have a rest before returning home again.

We had many different cases to deal with over the years. There was quite a lot of fraternizing with the Germans, as the maternity ward proved, but as the saying goes "c'est la guerre"! (that's war).

The German Officers were a bossy lot and tried to make everyone feel small.

We had all the cases of miscarriages to deal with on surgical ward, and had to put up with members of the forces visiting their girl friends and bringing all sorts of goodies for them.

One afternoon I was busy in the ward kitchen, getting patients' teas sorted out, when a huge Officer (why they were all so big I just don't know) marched in, holding a covered pie-dish which he gave to me saying: "You cook this for ... - it's for her tea." "What is it?" "It's bird, very good for her, I shoot blackbird, I clean, you cook, yes?" "Very well." "You do this?" "Oh yes." He watched as I popped it into the kitchen Aga, turned on his heel, with a "click", and walked back into the ward, feeling very pleased with himself. He was happier than I was!

When the visitors had left, I made sure I took this particular girl her tray myself. When she saw what was on her tray and asked what it was, I told her: "Your friend brought it in to me to cook for you to have for your tea, it's a blackbird which he shot especially for you!"

I just can't repeat what she said. Her face was quite a picture. The other patients were very amused by it all. Someone else was very pleased though - that was the ward cat, he certainly enjoyed his tea that day!

A local lady, a very well known personality, was admitted for minor surgery. She was put in the side ward. She was in hospital because she was going to die, or so she kept telling us. She had had major surgery some years previously which had been successful, but this little do, to her, was the last straw. Incidentally, it was nothing to do with her previous operation, but she kept telling us she was going to die.

Doctors and Nursing Staff all tried to reassure her, but no, she knew best and rang her bell every few minutes, night and day, always with a sad and sorrowful story. She was a very trying patient, thank goodness there weren't too many like her.

One day, on answering her bell, I was told: "Sit down, Nurse; I want to explain to you exactly what I want at my funeral, and I want you to promise me that my wishes will be carried out."

Oh, dear, I thought, here we go again. Luckily we were not too busy and I could spend a bit of time with her.

After writing down details of hymns and readings that she wanted for the service I promised to hand over the aforesaid details to whoever. This was all in a sealed envelope and placed in her locker. Before sealing it she suddenly said she didn't want anyone spending money on flowers for her grave. She just wanted a small bunch of wild daisies.

Needless to say she was discharged a few days after this, in good health, and lived for many more years. I never knew if she ever had her daisies or not.

On another occasion we had a special lady in the side ward who had such a lovely disposition. She always had a smile for everyone.

Before going off day duty we always checked all was well with each individual patient: pillows right, glass of water handy, all the little things that meant so much to a patient. When we got to this particular lady's bed, she'd say, with that lovely smile of hers, "You know what I want, don't you Nurse?" – Oh yes, we knew.

This lady had had a perineum repair and was terrified that she might move awkwardly during the night and do herself some damage. So, much to the amusement of the other ladies in the ward, we had to tie her knees together with bandage so that should she move in the night there would be no serious consequences.

Of course, we were only too pleased to oblige, amid a lot of ribbing. Here was one lady who would have a good night.

ANAESTHETICS

Everyone acts differently when coming out of an anaesthetic. Some can be very belligerent, some "happy as Larry", and some very tearful.

One farmer's wife, who was admitted one evening, had received a fractured clavicle and humerus after a nasty fall in the cows' stable.

Having visited the theatre to have everything sorted out, she was returned to the ward and then strapped up in a very uncomfortable looking position with her left arm in a Thomas' splint stretched out across a locker top to support it. She caused a great deal of amusement on coming around from anaesthetic, talking all the time. She had just brought the cows in for milking when she had the fall, so her mind was still on the care of the cows, and she was chatting away to Rosie and Bella, which with her uninjured hand she was very busy "milking".

Poor soul, she did feel embarrassed when the other patients told her how they had enjoyed "the show". Thankfully she took everything in good heart and was a very cheerful patient, and quite popular with the rest of the ward.

Making beds seemed to be an everlasting task, though it was good to look back down the ward and see everything neat and fresh looking. There were times when we just couldn't win with some patients. It didn't matter how much we tried, their bed just wouldn't look presentable, let alone comfortable.

This calls to mind a lady who was rather on the large side (to say the least). Because of her condition she was on a surgical bed; one that could be adjusted to suit the case.

There was a key to wind up the top of the base to form a back rest, and the middle part to make a support under the knees, which helped stop the patient sliding down the bed.

This lady was so large, every time she moved the whole bed became a mess. The top of the undersheet would slide down into a lump under her pillows; sometimes the pillows would go too. A lot of this was due to the horrible rubber sheeting which soon 'rucked' up.

Ordinarily we would lift the patient – one nurse standing on each side of the bed, supporting the patient's back with joined hands, and their other hands joined under the patient's knees, to give a 'lift' up the bed.

No way could we lift this lady, and often we'd stand on the back of the bed frame, two nurses together, grab the bottom sheet and pull like mad to get enough of the sheet to tuck it under the top end of the mattress, no easy task. Sometimes it worked and sometimes it didn't, like the time two colleagues attempting to do just this, had an unpleasant experience when the sheet split and they almost toppled out of the open window.

The saying goes, "variety is the spice of life". There was always plenty variety in "hospital life".

LIFE GOES ON

Life had to go on. Food was short and not very satisfying. It was the main topic of conversation.

A woman patient out on the balcony had to have a wound, which was not healing as it should, cauterized. I felt somewhat embarrassed when a woman I was attending to in the main ward remarked, "What a lovely smell, someone must be having roast beef for dinner!" Although we said, "No, no way," and gave some sort of explanation, I don't think we were believed. The patient was certain the smell was coming from the kitchen.

Thank goodness the lady having the cauterization never heard the remark.

THE WARD CAT

I must tell you the story about our ward cat. The one that had the blackbird for his tea.

He was first introduced to the domestics on women's ward. When we were trying to think of a suitable name for him "Gustie", who was an Austrian Jewish girl working at the hospital said: "We call him Churchill. He just like Churchill. He no good cat, he no catch mouse." So the name stuck.

Several weeks later I went to visit some friends. When I arrived there was a big discussion going on – rumour was rife. One was always greeted with "Have you heard this or that?"

As I walked in it was "Hello! Have you heard the latest about Mr. Churchill?" I thought, typical. "No, what's happened?" "He's broken his leg!" – "Really?" – "Yes, 'so and so' heard about it today."

I just doubled up with laughter. They all thought me mad, but I had the last laugh. When I was able to explain what I was laughing at, they had quite a surprise.

A couple of days previously our ward cat, Churchill, had got caught in a sliding door and had broken his leg. One of the Doctors and a Staff Nurse took pity on him and put his leg in plaster. My friends, now put in the picture, and understanding how very quickly rumour spreads, all had a good laugh. I wonder what our great man, Sir Winston, would have made of that little episode!

Just goes to show how hungry we were for news and how a little snippet overheard had become "Latest News headlines."

The story of Churchill the cat brings back very sad memories of that Jewish girl Gustie Spitz, the ward maid who christened him. She was a real character. I always got on well with her, though she really had no time for the English way of life and just couldn't get on with the language.

She was deported with two other Jewish girls, Marianne Grunfeld, who was working in another part of the island, and Theresa Steiner, who was Nursing with us. She was a very well respected Nurse, very good at her job, and well liked by all. She was a very refined girl and a brilliant musician. Many are the relaxing times we enjoyed in the recreation room listening to her playing the piano.

It greatly upset us all to hear that Nurse Steiner and Gustie were to be deported and the sight of the German Officers arriving to pick them up was very distressing. That was on 24th April 1942.

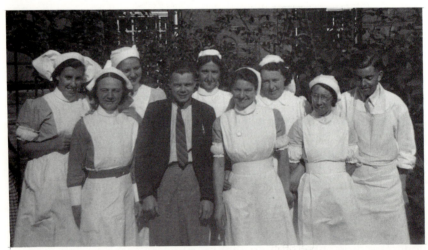

Nurse Steiner: back row between Sister and Male Nurse

They, along with Marianne Grunfeld, were taken to a concentration camp on 27th April 1942. They were taken from St. Malo, along with other Jews, to the Drancy camp, then on to Auschwitz on the 23rd July 1942. It is believed that they died on that day.

We didn't know what had happened to them until well after the war had ended. We all had a good idea as to what they had gone to, and were horrified at the thought that those girls we had worked with and known had ended their lives in such a way. I cannot put into words what I felt and indeed still do feel about it all, as do many of my old colleagues.

THE CHILDREN'S WARD

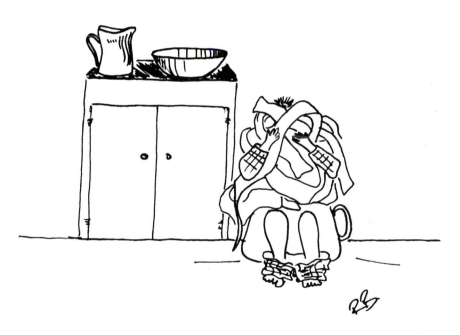

"Nursey, Nursey, can't see me!"

I well remember a little fair-haired lad of 2-2½ years old, who was with us on Women's Ward (before we had a Children's Ward). He had had a mishap with boiling water and had received burns to his arm. He was a lively little chap and quite bright.

Some of the nurses weren't very happy because he always wet his bed at night. While I was on duty I made a habit of lifting the little sleepy head out every night. Consequently he was dry every morning – to me that was the simple answer. I don't think the little fellow even knew he'd been out of bed, let alone performed for me.

Every morning when issuing the patients with their bowls of water to wash, I'd have him "helping" me. We got on like a house on fire. He was so happy trotting around and, as it was only his arm that was burned, it did him good to run around provided we watched his dressings covered the burns and that he didn't knock himself.

With all the running around I'd try to pot him on time. One morning, having left him on the pot while I did something else, I came back to see a whole heap of toilet paper from which came a lot of giggles. The little scamp had reached for the toilet roll and had had a grand time pulling it all out over himself.

He looked so cheeky sitting there on the pot, two bright little eyes peeping amongst the paper. "Nursey, Nursey, you can't see me!"

Another time I gave him a toilet roll to take to one of the patients. Up he trotted to the bed. "Here y'are, Grannie, and make no mess!" He certainly kept the women amused.

We eventually got a Children's Ward. What had once been the inmates dormitory was turned into a ward, the inmates having been moved to another part of the hospital.

Working on Children's Ward was another interesting experience. The kids were wonderful to look after. We had all age groups to care for, from small babies to about eight years old, with various ailments. Some were suffering from malnutrition, general illnesses, bronchitis, pneumonia, accidents, broken limbs, burns, also general operations such as tonsillectomy, appendectomy, and often dental cases. Quite a variety!

The Sister in charge was a great character, a dedicated disciplinarian who loved the children. The children loved her and responded to her and her skills.

Food was pretty basic, but always made to look attractive to the little patients. Sister would visit the kitchens every morning and try to get a variety of foods for her important little people. One thing she insisted on was fresh vegetables and would badger the person preparing the vegetables for some pieces of raw root vegetables that she could give to the children to chew. They looked forward to their carrots and bits of mangel-wurzel.

She always endeavoured to make the children's stay a happy one, and all her staff were trained to give plenty of cuddles, and to read lovely bed-time stories, which we enjoyed as much as the kids. Goodness knows where the story books came from. Then there would be sing-songs, which we'd all join in. Nursery Rhymes were favourite of course. And there were special treats too. There were occasions when we had to be quiet naturally, according to what type of cases we had on the ward, and there were some very sad circumstances at times.

However, believe it or not, we had a pair of song-birds who spent a lot of time on the balcony when it was fine enough for them. The two boys (about seven or eight years) with bad burns, had lovely voices and Sister always encouraged them. They could let off a bit of steam out there.

They knew "The Trolley Song" and "Mares eat oats and Does eat oats" right the way through, and other songs. Where had they learnt these songs? Sister had taught them. Many things were picked up on Sister's hidden radio (not in the hospital). We knew now for sure that the snippets of news she let slip at times were the genuine thing from the B.B.C. Sister was living in her own little house about five minutes away from the hospital.

The boys loved having their beds outdoors and would call out to the workers and ambulance personnel as they went by. Everyone knew them and would give them a cheery word. Both boys were some of the first to be sent to the U.K. for treatment after Liberation.

Christmas on Children's Ward was a happy experience to say the least. The weeks of our two songsters practising their carols didn't mar their actual Christmas Day renderings. They were sweet kids as were the rest of the little patients on this ward.

For many of the island's children it was a hard time. Santa had a very difficult job to find enough gifts. However the Christmas I spent with them on that ward wasn't too bad.

My brother-in-law had been very busy making children's toys in wood for some time, to make a little extra for his family at the festive season. At that time there was a lot of Black Marketeering and if you had the wherewithal you could get the goods. However, my brother-in-law made lorries and skittles among other things. I was so thrilled to present Sister with some of these wooden toys, with his compliments, so with second-hand books and homemade bits and pieces Santa made a pretty good job of his visit. Then the parents brought little gifts too, so all in all the kids had a good time.

Another Nurse and myself spent most of the day entertaining the children as best we could, as they were all bedridden.

One thing they did enjoy was to see their two Nurses down on the floor playing skittles. One side of the ward cheered one of us and the other side stuck up for the other Nurse. There was a lot of laughing and shouting. The skittles were standing at the end of the ward across the doorway, and we were aiming with the balls to knock as many as possible over.

Suddenly, the door opened and in walked Matron! Needless to say we felt such fools, down on our hands and knees scrambling after skittle balls, creating a heck of a racket. To our amazement Matron got down on her knees and joined the fun. I don't know who enjoyed it most. Matron spent the rest of the afternoon with us and we all finished up with a sing-song.

The patients were tired but happy and it was a bit difficult to get them to settle that evening, but, with one or two favourite stories, with them tucked up, their eyelids soon began to droop. It had been a grand day for them, as all the happy little slumbering faces proved.

Matron often caught me out, doing something daft. I well remember one Friday morning, in particular. Friday was "teeth and tonsils" day, two very messy jobs in theatre. This particular day I had to take a little 4-year-old boy up to theatre for a tonsillectomy.

As there had been some delay in theatre, I had to amuse young Billy until they were ready for him. I was sitting outside the anaesthetic room with him on my knee acting out "Two little Dickie Birds sitting on a wall", with bits of plaster stuck on my fingers as the birds. Billy and I were so engrossed we didn't realize we were being watched. He was repeating after me, "Two little dickie birds sitting on a wall, one named Peter and one named Paul. Fly away Peter, fly away Paul. Come back Peter, come back Paul!" I was busy enacting the flyaway and come back bits, over and over again, when a voice behind me said, "How do you do that, Nurse? I can't see how it's done. I've never seen that before."

So once Billy was off my hands, I had to teach Matron the trick. I felt really silly and was glad that I didn't have to explain to Sister why I had been so long off the ward. She was satisfied that theatre was running a bit late.

The more I got to know Matron the more I admired her. Although she could be very dignified and severe, she could certainly treat one as an equal at times.

Night-duty on Children's Ward was a bit lonely. One coped single-handed, but soon got used to it, though it could be a bit eerie at times. Duty Sister always checked during the night that everything was alright, and another Nurse would take over for meal-time when we'd join the others.

It was at times difficult to keep awake when there was no one else to talk to. However, if there was a babe on two-hourly feeds or one of the children needed some sort of treatment, things wouldn't be so trying.

One night-duty down there was a bit scary. There was a man missing from the annexe where there were some mentally ill men. It was pretty worrying to be alone on the ward knowing that the man could quite easily come up the fire escape. Thankfully nothing occurred and he was found first thing next morning safe and well. No one had dared search away from the hospital areas during the hours of curfew.

One good remedy for keeping awake was a good splash in the face under the cold water tap. It helped a lot.

Having to go on to another ward for meals at night meant a walk from the Children's Ward which took one up on to the balcony of the female ward, past the Burns and T.B. patients. It was quite a tricky walk in the dark owing to the black-out. One advantage was the fact that there was a rail at one side where it overlooked the yard below.

Imagine the fright one Nurse got when walking from Children's Ward in the middle of the night to go for her dinner. Walking quietly and as carefully as possible, feeling for the rail, she put her hand on a head of hair. Knowing there was a woman in the side ward opposite who was suicidal she really thought that the woman had hanged herself over the balcony, and dashed into the ward only to find the woman tucked up in bed and a Nurse on vigil at her bedside. The Nurse felt silly, fancy forgetting there was always someone night and day with that patient. O.K. but, if <u>she</u> was alright, <u>who</u> was that out there?

Both Nurses went out somewhat scared, wondering who or what they'd find and risked having a bit of light shining through the ward door so that they could see what they were investigating. There they found a *floor mop* that one of the ward maids had washed and left out to dry! They were both glad of a cup of tea after that shock. Even though it was only <u>bramble</u> tea, it was <u>very</u> welcome.

Next morning the ward maid responsible was told of the fright she had given them. Poor woman was quite upset at first, then they all had a good laugh. After all, the Nurse did manage to eat her dinner later, so there was no harm done.

One got to expect all sorts of things when on night-duty, particularly when a certain male nurse was on nights, as he was an incorrigible practical joker.

More will be revealed about him later.

THEATRE WORK

Theatre work was another world. I must admit it was a world I thoroughly enjoyed. Hard, tiring work, but so very interesting.

The Matron of surgical ward acted as the Surgeon's assistant in all operations be it night or day. The theatre was her domain. I'm sure that had any of the surgeons or doctors collapsed during an operation she would have just calmly taken over and finished the operation, and made an excellent job of it too.

Many a time when a young, less experienced, Doctor was operating and seemed to hesitate, she would in a very subtle way, mention she had seen this particular operation done a certain way. Many a hint was dropped and taken up in a very discreet manner. Of course <u>we</u> were too inexperienced to realize the Doctor was being helped or so, we hoped, <u>he</u> thought.

The theatre staff consisted of the surgeon, his assistant (Matron), the anaesthetist (choice of three), one theatre nurse, and the nurse from the patient's ward, who would assist the theatre nurse. That was for standard operations. If it should be a major operation, then we'd have a Sister or Staff Nurse extra.

Having done some theatre duties on and off from the wards, I was able to learn a lot from the theatre Nurse on duty, experiencing preparation procedures, learning which instruments were to be sterilized for which operation, and the preparing of instrument trolleys and trays etc., which caps and gowns for whom (some Doctors were very particular about caps, gowns and gloves), helping to gown up Doctors, learning what to do and what <u>not</u> to do. There was so much to remember.

During the operation one had to be alert all the time, ready to mop a surgeon's brow when needed, change positions of the table and lights, check and count the swabs before and after, we didn't want any left in the patient, did we?

Once the last stitch was in, and the patient had been wheeled back into the ward, it was cleaning and clearing up time. At times pretty straight-forward, at others there was plenty mess to clean up. I won't go into details. It was quite a hectic life.

As you will appreciate we had no lectures or schooling for any of our work. It was all practical. We did do our own bit of swotting if we could get hold of the appropriate books. The staff on Medical Wards did have lectures, given by the Resident Doctor. Matron had a very good system going, in that we all got the chance of a variety of work. There were Male surgical day and night duties, also work on female and children's wards, and a spell of theatre work. Everyone did the varied shifts and as time went on we became more generally experienced. Those who weren't happy in one field were encouraged in another.

One day when clearing up after a case in theatre, Matron, who always attended to her own side of things and usually chatted whilst doing whatever, suddenly said, "Do I upset you Nurse, if I shout at you during an operation?" "Not really Matron, if I have done something I shouldn't have, well, I do take notice, but if on the other hand we are in a tricky situation and I know you're worried, well, no, it's like water off a duck's back. You can shout all you like." I don't think I would have said so much had I stopped to consider it. Luckily she saw the funny side of things. "I'm so pleased you're honest with me," she said, "so many of my Nurses seem to be terrified of me when I shout."

We had a good understanding after that little discussion and many a time later when things seemed to be going wrong in theatre and she'd shout for this or that, I only had to look at her and see her eyes twinkling behind her mask. We understood each other.

Some of the operations were very interesting, and it was a privilege to watch the skill of one particular surgeon. As he got to know who was genuinely interested, he would get us nearer to the table and take a lot of trouble to explain what he was doing and why, making sure we understood what he was talking about. He was the one surgeon who never ever walked out of theatre without thanking us all individually for our help. He was a very clever, dedicated and skilful man, who spent what spare time he had studying so that he could use his skill to the best of his abilities. A true gentleman.

We had many appendectomies over the years. One that I remember well was a girl in her teens who had been rushed in diagnosed as acute appendix and was operated on straight away. When the surgeon had got through to the necessary area, he had a little laugh and was highly amused at something. Matron, who was assisting, was having a giggle too, so very unlike them both in the middle of surgery. We two Nurses looked at each other wondering what was going on. Then Doctor told us to come and see what he had found. There was the appendix well and truly exposed, but looking quite healthy. The actual pain that poor girl had been suffering was caused by a brown kidney bean lodged in a small cavity near the appendix. Beans at that time were a much appreciated diet when you could get them.

To get back to this poor girl, the bean was carefully removed and so too was the appendix. As it is not an essential piece of equipment in our bodies, the surgeon deemed it wise to remove it just the same. At least it would never cause her any trouble at a future date.

A senior Nurse and I always enjoyed watching this particular surgeon's work and were fascinated by his skill and the speed with which he worked on the straight-forward cases. For a bit of fun, unknown to him, we started timing him on the appendectomy. From the first incision to the final stitch, if I remember correctly, it was ten minutes for a straight-forward job. Somehow he discovered what we were up to and often tried to better his time. I must hastily add that by no means was there ever any risk to the patient. He was too caring a man for that. I don't think he did improve his time, not when I was in theatre.

Amputations were not a very pleasant job, but we all knew that these things were done solely in the patient's interest and well-being. Leg amputations were a very heavy job and we all needed to be on the alert the whole time, hoping not to cause the patient too much stress. The anaesthetist too played a very important part in all cases. Everybody needed very quick reactions every time. But amputations were a worry to all the team. What with the heat of the theatre and our poor diet, it was extremely tiring for all. We felt heavily committed to the well-being of the patient who was going to have so much to face up to, the adjusting to the loss of a limb and the pain to be endured. It takes a very brave person to fight through it all.

In many cases it was difficult to know what types of catgut to use as replacements were almost impossible. Some equipment and medicines were brought over from France, but not always exactly what was needed. Subsequently the wrong type or size of catgut had to be used, thus causing many problems with the sutures. A wound wouldn't heal and it often led to septic wounds, the stitches causing a lot of discomfort.

That meant the patient having to submit to receiving hot fomentations to draw out the pus which had accumulated. Not very nice, particularly with stamina so low. It was very unpleasant for the patient.

With the assortment of cases, the different operations, such as hernias, gall stones, bladder problems, hysterectomies, ovarian troubles, perenium repairs, appendectomies, mastectomies, various abdominal cases, ears, nose and throat, plus fractures to set and put in plaster, cuts and tears to be repaired and stitched, and on Friday mornings tonsillectomies and teeth, there was always something of interest going on.

When there was no surgery being carried out, there were always instruments to be cleaned and prepared for sterilization, plus swabs of various types and towels to be checked. Drums to be packed and an assortment of receptacles and receivers cleaned and put in the sterilizer. Everything had to be ready for the next case, which could be at any time of the day or night.

I think the most exciting cases were the Caesarean sections. There was always that feeling of anticipation and excitement as Mum was wheeled into theatre and carefully lifted on to the table.

The surgeon, with such care, would make the first incision, and continue the approach until the time would come when we'd see for the first time ever that little babe floating in the "sac". A wonderful sight. In those days the incision was right down the centre of the tummy, so we all had a clear view. Then it was "action stations". With what seemed a flick of the scalpel, we'd all be paddling in water, but no one noticed that, all eyes were on this new life which was held up for all to see and carefully checked, then passed over to the waiting Sister to be well wrapped up snug and warm in a crib. Everyone was happy as lusty cries came from the new arrival.

Now it was all attention on Mum, to get her sorted out, cleaned and stitched up, and got back into the ward as soon as possible. And later, it was so rewarding to see a very proud Mum sitting up in the ward nursing the new babe.

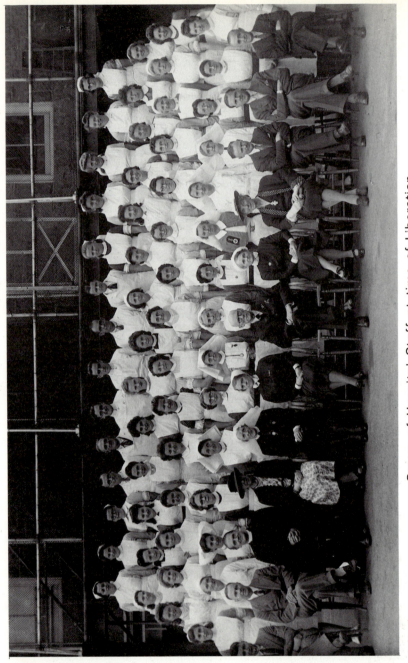

Group of Hospital Staff at time of Liberation

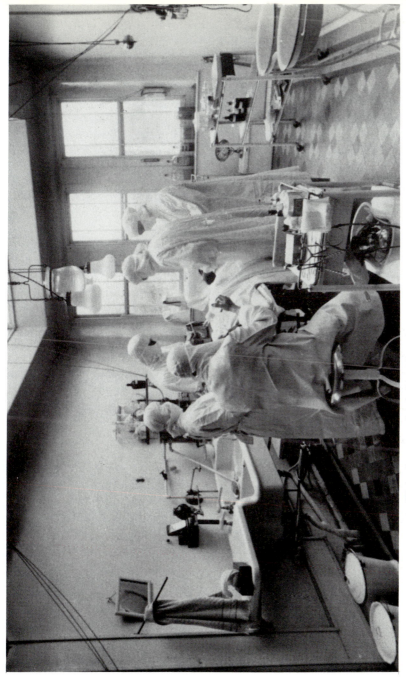

This is an old 'photo' taken in 1920s or 1930s
We worked in this theatre which had had many improvements by the 1940s

I've said very little about anaesthetists who did such good and very responsible work too. A nurse always accompanied the patient into the anaesthetic room, ready to assist if needed.

Accident cases tended to be somewhat antagonistic and fought against the anaesthetic. One had to be so careful that they didn't do themselves more injury. On one occasion, a man who had been injured in an accident, suddenly sat bolt upright on the stretcher and landed a punch on the nurse in attendance. She just flew backwards across the room. Fortunately the porters were on hand and were able to restrain the patient until the anaesthetic took over. I'm sure that man would have been most embarrassed had he known what he had done.

These cases had to be watched closely as they came out of the anaesthetic too, as they could do a lot of damage to themselves. Once they were aware of what was what, there was no more trouble. It is surprising how anaesthetic affects some more than others.

Friday mornings were very busy and messy. Tonsil-lectomies were done first. I always felt sorry for the children who had to go through such an uncomfortable time. Next would be the dental cases. The dentists came out to the hospital to do these extractions. They'd work very quickly with their patient under a light anaesthetic.

One particular dentist was a nuisance to say the least. The Nurse in attendance had the job of holding a receptacle near at hand for the dentist to drop the teeth in, but this dentist worked so fast yanking out teeth and with a flick of his wrist would send teeth flying all over the place. If you got in the line of fire, too bad. I can laugh now, but he was so arrogant, no use asking him to drop the teeth into the receiver "please!" When he was finished it was a case of "hunt the teeth." They had been flicked in every direction and there were teeth and blood splashes everywhere. It took quite some time to clean up after him. Once the morning was through, the theatre was closed for the week-end to enable the cleaners to have a good go at it all. That, of course, was unless there was an emergency.

The theatre cleaner in charge was a middle-aged lady. She was always ready and waiting to start on "her theatre", or "my theatre" as she called it. We weren't out of the door that she was starting to clean. She got so frustrated when she sometimes found a tooth that we'd missed. "Those Nurses", they never did their job right, and they'd mucked up her brasses that had been splashed with blood.

To give her credit, she took great pride in her work. The theatre would be absolutely spotless, with brasses, taps, pipes and sterilizers "gleaming". And the tiles and floor spotless.

As the theatre was a very confined area, it was the ideal spot to catch up on the latest news and gossip without fear of anyone overhearing.

Once the actual operations were over and everything had been checked and given the O.K., it was time for a little gossip, during the clearing-up procedures. Everyone had something to contribute. Having worked with the Doctors and Senior Staff for so long, although we held them all in high esteem, we were not in "awe" of them. We were as one happy family when work and responsibilities were over.

The fact that we had to make our own fun and entertainment did help us all to get to know one another quite well socially, but we never took advantage of the fact when on duty.

The Doctors would occasionally exchange news of their families who were all in the U.K. The only news they got was a short message through the Red Cross. These were always a great delight to us all, even though they consisted of so few words and came infrequently, having taken quite a while to come through. Everyone shared their messages with whoever showed interest.

One of the Nursing Staff's parents and sister were deported to Germany. She stayed on as she was in an essential position. Before her family departed they had got together and between them contrived a code, which was an ideal way of passing on news. As you can well imagine we were always longing for her to receive her Red Cross messages, longing to know what they contained and learned quite a bit about what was happening the other side of the Channel. They in their turn were, I'm sure, glad to know what was going on here. We were, one and all, hungry for news of any sort.

— — — — —

Until the Germans had found themselves a place to use as a hospital, at the beginning of the occupation, when needed, they'd use our operating theatre with their surgeons and staff, of course. We had to look after their patients until they were well enough to be moved on. There weren't many cases, which was just as well, because our lads were not very happy to have Germans on the ward. Thank goodness those circumstances didn't last long. The Germans soon got themselves sorted out.

Another incident worth mentioning was the fact that we had a couple of R.A.F. lads with us for a few days. They had crashed into the sea off the north coast of the island, swam ashore, and were captured by the Germans and eventually brought to us for treatment and a check-up. They were then taken away as prisoners of war as soon as they were well enough.

One of them left some personal item and a message with one of the Nurses, for her to pass on if and when she could. What it was or for whom, no one else knew for the Nurse never told anyone.

TOPIC OF CONVERSATION

Food was a favourite topic of conversation. It was in short supply and not very satisfying. It must have been a nightmare for the caterers to keep everyone going.

There came a time when it was pretty awful having to take such poor meals to patients who needed feeding up or should have been tempted with some little delicacy. All they got was a couple of spoonfuls of mashed swede or just soggy spinach. Some would say, "Keeping all the good food for the Nurses are they?" Many just couldn't or wouldn't believe that what they had for meals was what we got too, and we had to work for several hours on it.

For 'afters' it was generally something milky. For quite a time it was macaroni pudding but with a difference. Somebody had discovered some sacks of macaroni in a warehouse and had passed the lot on to the hospital. Down in the kitchen at this time there were huge cauldrons of water with the macaroni soaking in them. Floating on top of the water were literally hundreds of dead maggots. The kitchen porter had the job of skimming them off the top. But by the time the puddings had been made more maggots appeared from inside the tubes of macaroni. However, what didn't fatten filled, at least what we saw could be left on the side of the plate. You just didn't have to think about what might have still been in the macaroni you'd swallowed.

One thing that was good and helped us all, patients and staff, was soup. There always seemed to be a good supply of that, and it was something the patients could enjoy. It was not as rich as we'd have liked, but it went down well.

We were receiving rations of horse meat from France. It was very coarse and tough, but better than no meat at all. No doubt the horse bones helped to make good stock for soups. For a change we'd have mince in gravy. I hate to think <u>what</u> it was that <u>was</u> minced, still, we did survive. "What the eye didn't see!"

Breakfast was usually something called porridge, made with various types of meal and cereal, some of it looked very much like the meal given to pigs and smelt like it! Other times it would be thicker and quite appetizing, apart from all the husks that were in it. Table manners were pretty well non-existent, everyone fishing out what we could that was indigestible and just swallowing the remainder.

The bread, too, was very heavy and coarse and full of husks, what little we had of it. It was very grey in colour. We were each given a small ration to last the week. If you ate it all in one go that was your bad luck, no more until next week.

Tea time was when we needed our bread. On the dining-room table there would be, maybe, a couple of large platters with lettuce leaves, so it was honeymoon sandwiches that day (let us alone). Next day it could be "sweaty feet" sandwiches, that was Camembert cheese from France which was so ripe it was running out of the boxes, but it did <u>taste</u> good and made a change. Another day it could be sugar beet treacle. It was something to go on the bread, that is if you had any left.

Supper time it was mostly soup.

Adjacent to the Nurses' Dining-Room was the Senior Staff Dining-Room, i.e. Matrons and Sisters. At the time when food was getting shorter and shorter and less and less appetizing, the Nursing Staff put in a complaint. Everyone was on strict rations, so, why was it the Nurses were existing on the same food as the patients with little or no variations and yet delicious smells were wafting in from next door?

After many discussions and threats of strikes, we were addressed by a member of the board and told that we would have a Senior member, either a Matron or Sister joining us for meals in the future. They took it in turns. It was something I suppose. But we all felt we had been treated like children and we <u>had</u> made our point. I must admit the Senior Staff were very sympathetic with us and even joined in with counting the maggots. They spent one week each with us, and ate whatever we did. To be quite honest not one of us would have carried out the threat of striking. We knew it was the Germans to blame. One just had to let it be known that we were not willing to be treated as 'under-dogs'.

It all sounds very childish now, and next door still had their little extras. We had stated our case. We were all in the same boat and we just had to make the best of things . . .

Until that wonderful day when the Red Cross Ship, the Vega, arrived with a supply of Red Cross Parcels.

That's another story that I shall tell you later.

— — — — —

One of the Doctors enjoyed fishing. His way of relaxing. (There were one or two areas free from mines).

Matron was in charge of theatre and woe betide anyone who did anything they shouldn't. She knew every instrument, dressing, etc. that there was in that theatre down to every bit of catgut which she guarded.

This Doctor often asked for little bits of catgut for his lines, but she was adamant. If he so much as looked towards those jars, she'd be on at him. "It's no use you looking like that Doctor, you're just <u>not</u> having any. I've got my patients to think of!" – She was in her rights, no one knew when or if we'd get a fresh supply, or, what it would be like if we did get some. All this silly bantering added a bit of fun to the day.

OCTOBER 1943

There had been a great battle in the Channel and many British Navy personnel lost their lives. Many bodies were washed up on our shores.

The Germans gave permission for them to be buried at the Foulon Cemetery with full honours, and Islanders were allowed to attend. Many turned up to pay their respects to the men from H.M.S. Charybdis. All walks of life were represented, including a group of us Nurses in uniform.

It was a lovely bright and sunny day. There were such crowds of islanders there, that the Germans were not that pleased to see such loyalty.

I will not dwell on it, so much has already been written about it.

HOME MADE ENTERTAINMENT

As I have already said, we made our own entertainment. We had our Social Committee and endeavoured to have a good evening's entertainment once a month. Sometimes it would be a musical evening. We had quite a lot of talent amongst the staff.

Around Christmas-time we'd hold a special dance, when each member of the staff was allowed to invite a partner and, because of the curfew it was always arranged for the partners to stay overnight; sleeping on mattresses with blankets on an empty ward floor or in the recreation room, wherever space could be found.

Often we held our own variety shows, which were always great fun – the staff of each floor competing against one another. The Doctors too, always did their bit at these shows, and enjoyed it all.

One Doctor was a gifted violinist and he was accompanied by one of the Nurses who was an excellent pianist. Between them they contributed a lot towards very enjoyable musical evenings.

There would also be the various duets, solos and group singing. Sometimes light music, other times classical.

Two of the Doctors, who were great friends, would without fail entertain us with their solos, the one always trying to outdo the other. They put their heart and soul into their renderings of a large variety of songs. They, like many others, had wives and families in the U.K. but they never seemed to let things get them down, one seldom saw them anything but cheerful, though I'm sure they must have had their moments of doubt and worry. They were both very popular with their patients, and gave of their best.

We had three Sisters on the surgical wards and, not a concert went by without three of the Doctors acting out skits, which they wrote themselves, about the Sisters. These we always enjoyed as the lyrics were always so well written and topical. They dressed up as Sisters with wigs and starched caps.

One song I've never forgotten or, should I say, part of one. The lyrics were very good, picking up many of the expressions and mannerisms of the Sisters. After all the patter and humour they finished up with "And what's more, we are British to the back-bone!" And with this they turned around together and with their backs to us, bent down and threw their skirts over their heads displaying three "Union Jacks" across their backsides.

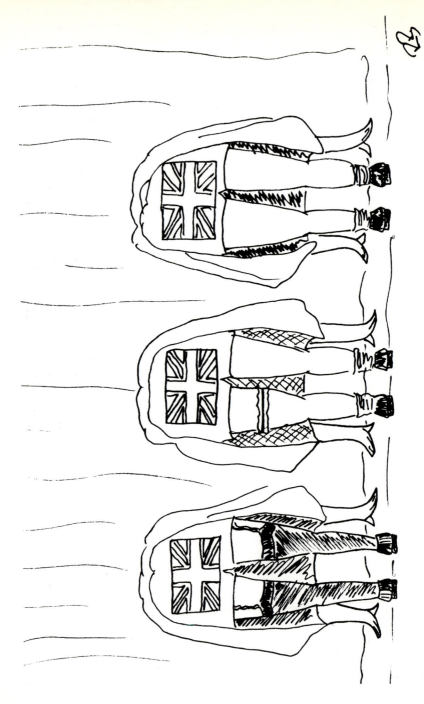

The three patriots!

Anything British, or red white and blue, meant so much to us, as it was *"verboten*". (The Germans wouldn't have been impressed).

Some of the Nurses were good dancers, so we had "taps" and other costume dances, which were very well performed. One Nurse was an excellent "Burlington Bertie", dressed the part, with top hat, monocle and cane.

Another Nurse was Jazz mad and could also rattle out any tune you wanted, all played by ear. There were also humorous recitations and monologues. You name it and someone could do it. It was all for a good carefree evening.

The duet I remember well was one that a colleague and I performed. It was a humorous song, "Oh Henry!" "O Sara"! about a farmer's lad and his milkmaid. We dressed in appropriate costumes, my milkmaid looking very sweet and innocent in her floral dress, apron and bonnet. Myself in "bib & brace" overalls, check shirt and straw hat, carrying a hay-rake and chewing a straw. The chorus was really "lovey dovey" with Sara and Henry gazing into each other's eyes; how we didn't break down laughing in the middle of that song I'll never know. Fifty years on is a long time to recall the words, but I do remember something about having, "a piece of string tied around my thumb to recollect you see, to ask you, Sara dear, if you would marry me." Then the chorus of "Oh Henry!" and "Oh Sara!" with lots of sighs.

It must have been O.K. because, whenever we saw a certain Doctor later he wouldn't let us forget it. He always told 'Sara' he would never have thought she had it in her to act as she did, and he often called her "Sara". With me, it was a long time before I lived it down too. On meeting this particular Doctor at the ward door to accompany him on his rounds, as was usual, I greeted him with "Good Morning Doctor", he answered by saying, "Good Morning Nurse" (then, under his breath) "And how is Henry this morning?"

He was my sister's G.P. and at the time of her first confinement he attended her. This particular day, 19th October 1943, I had just come out of the anaesthetic room when Doctor came running down the stairs from Labour Ward. "Oh, Nurse, I'm so glad I've found you," he said, "I thought you'd like the pleasure of 'phoning your brother-in-law, to let him know Mother and Baby are both well." Then with his head on the side, "But it's not a Henry"! What a way to be told I had a niece.

That all happened many years ago. "Sara" and I are still in touch. Although we worked on different floors, living in the same digs we got to know each other very well, we shared our joys and our sorrows. These days when we get together we share many memories and many many laughs. I shall never forget the enjoyable times we spent together. Thank you "Sara".

— — — — —

Our Matron was of the old school She had served abroad during the 1914-18 War in Salonika. She was always very smart, immaculately dressed, her uniform perfect in every way, but, she had one funny little habit, and those Doctors found out about it and weren't going to let her get away with anything.

They frequently teased her about her service abroad. They wrote a song about her, when she was young and flirting with the officers sitting under the palm trees, etc. She was always ready for a laugh, and took it all in good part. We really enjoyed it all. Then they came to the "crunch"

"And what's more <u>we</u> know where Matron keeps her hankie!" her little aforesaid habit. She kept her hankie tucked into the edge of her knicker elastic.

The Doctors didn't get away with all their skits "scot free". Some of the Nurses turned the tables on them.

One Doctor loved his fishing, a couple of others were sports' fanatics. The girls, dressed appropriately, gave them some of their own medicine. They had written several verses about the Doctors and their pastimes. One dressed in oilskins and rods, another in cricket whites, and one in other sports gear, I can't remember what. At that time the Doctors were cycling more as petrol was very scarce, so another Nurse, dressed in a smart suit, a trilby hat, and carrying a brief case, joined in the chorus by ringing a cycle bell with much enthusiasm. I only wish I could remember the words of their songs. One in particular was set to Widdecombe Fair, with the chorus of Doctors' names finishing with "and old Doctor ..... and all!".

Trying to think of something different for the concerts was becoming difficult. Then a Sister in our group remembered something she had done during her training years. We thought it was an excellent idea. "A mock orchestra!" Everyone in our group rallied round to find suitable instruments and attire. We finished up with: piano, violins, viola, 'cello and big bass, miming to an orchestral piece which was recorded.

As the curtain opened the "orchestra" was already playing. There were the violinists, blond girls in black evening dresses; the pianist was Sister, with short dark hair and wearing an evening suit; the 'cello and big bass were also played by dark haired girls in evening suits, and very smart they all looked too. Then, of course, there was the conductor, a tail coat, bristling whiskers, powdered hair (yours truly).

We had a lovely time "playing" the "Blue Danube" and it went down very well. Then unknown to us, the male Nurse whom we had trusted with the gramophone, decided to turn the record over and we found ourselves playing "Tales from Vienna Woods", which we had not rehearsed. It was all good fun.

Sister had always fancied herself as a concert pianist and very well she acted the part. Though I bet her hands were sore after thumping away on the piano lid.

Staff Nurse, on the bass, got carried away too, and would suddenly twirl the bass at an exciting moment. The blessed thing was bigger than her. It was hilarious.

— — — —

In the early years we had a mixed hospital hockey team of Doctors, Sisters and Nurses. We played against teams from Banks, The Essential Commodities Committee's team and The Guernsey Hockey Team. It was all good exercise and was something to do.

There came a time, though, when it was deemed to be too strenuous for us, plus the fact that many players were getting more and more minor injuries. So we abandoned the hockey team – two or three of the Nurses had received black eyes whilst playing and Matron thought it was very bad to have nurses working on the wards displaying black eyes. Of course, she was right. We were there to nurse not to <u>be</u> nursed.

A few days later, much to our surprise and, dare I say, some amusement, Matron entered the ward to do her usual rounds sporting a beautiful black eye. How we kept straight faces while escorting her around the ward I do not know.

It turned out that there had been an emergency during the night and Matron, as always, was called on to attend the theatre. Some special splints were needed for the case. The splint cupboard was on the floor that Matron had to pass on her way down from her room. On seeing a Nurse struggling with splints, Matron went to help her sort out what was needed. Unfortunately there were some bed pulleys standing nearby, one swung round and caught Matron in the eye. It must have been very painful for her and could have been much worse.

I'm ashamed to say we still found it really funny after the way we had all been told off for playing such a rough game as hockey and getting injured. Thankfully she did see the funny side of it too.

– – – –

The dances were varied, evening wear, fancy dress, or just casual, according to the time of the year.

For the evening wear there was quite an assortment of gowns that appeared, some of the staff had their own old faithful long dresses. Remember we had to use just whatever we had at the time of the occupation, no slipping into town to buy a new gown. There was a considerable amount of borrowing and lending done too.

One of the Doctors was very generous and loaned several of his wife's gowns (his wife was in the U.K.), so those who didn't have a suitable long dress were able to borrow one of these. I wonder what that Doctor felt seeing others in his wife's gowns. Was he thinking of his dear wife far away in the U.K.?

Everyone made a great effort to "dress up" and make the whole thing go with a swing. Nurses who could play the piano took it in turn to accompany the dancers. The male nurses joined in at times with drums and, or, piano-accordion. Then there was always the trusty old gramophone. Oh! we did ourselves proud! The patients near enough to the recreation room to hear some of the music enjoyed it too.

We had great fun with the Fancy Dress dances. These would cause quite a lot of puzzlement while masks were on. It's very surprising how you can work close to someone for so long, yet, if they didn't give a clue, what with costume and mask, you were often at a loss as to who it was.

I was caught out by one of the Doctors who was dressed as a Sister, in a beautiful wig and loads of make-up. I knew it was a Doctor, but which one? He changed his voice and kept me guessing for quite some time. By eliminating the other Doctors, I finally came to a decision and knew who it was before the unmasking. He had many of us fooled. I wonder where he got his high heeled shoes from. He did have rather large feet.

Two other Doctors turned up as the Heavenly Twins and very well they looked too, dressed in theatre gowns and socks, a lovely pair of wings, a halo bobbing over their heads, and each carrying a harp. They caused a few laughs. At a later dance they came as "V2", dressed to look like Jews, walking about together with "V2" displayed on their backs.

One young chap came as "The New Order". At the time we were still getting more orders from the Kommandant, very silly and petty things. So this bright lad decided to come as "The New Order". He had all his clothes on back to front, trousers, shirt with tie down his back, jacket also buttoned down his back, then a large trilby hat back to front on his head, which made him look ridiculous. All very cleverly worked out.

We had the usual assortment of gypsies, pirates, clowns and all the rest of it. Another Doctor really amused us (wicked that we were). He was something of an exhibitionist and I'm afraid we used to take "the micky" in everyday life. He turned up as "Prince Charming" in doublet and hose, with a large feather in his velvet cap. It made our day to see him thus arrayed in all his glory. He thought he was just "it" in his gorgeous costume. Much more refined than all our home made efforts.

Still, a good time was had by all, the only thing missing was refreshments. Rations wouldn't run to that. Though I must say that some of the dancers were "happy". My guess is someone had spent a bit on the "Black Market" and thus kept up their "spirits".

I often wonder where we found all our energy, being short of nourishing foods and working long and hard hours. We still managed to have a good time, everyone was so friendly, like one big happy family. Everyone was in the same boat, irrespective of class. All islanders were just waiting and longing to be free of the 'Jack-boot'.

— — — — —

Duties on Women's Surgical were never uneventful. We experienced all sorts.

The suicidal lady I mentioned before was a very unfortunate case. When the Germans ordered that all English-born residents had to be deported to Germany, naturally there was panic among many of the people in the islands who were in this category.

This lady and her husband from one of the other islands had made a pact. Rather than be deported, he would shoot her first and then himself. Unfortunately, or maybe fortunately, according to how you look at it, he hadn't killed her, but had succeeded in killing himself. So she was admitted in a very poor condition with gun-shot wounds. The fact that she had had to be transferred from another island to Guernsey didn't help. The surgeons dealt successfully with the gun-shot wounds, but, of course, the mental anguish was not so easily dealt with. She was with us for a long time.

We had many varying sad cases to deal with over the years. A doctor who had been on the island for only a short period of time before the occupation, was running a private practice. One young girl went to him for help and, I'm sorry to say, this so-called doctor performed an abortion on this poor girl. Consequently she was admitted to hospital in a very ill condition. Sadly after a lot of suffering, that girl passed away. The man responsible for her death was charged and imprisoned for many years. He deserved all he got, having caused the death of a lovely girl, and so much anguish and pain to her family. Thank goodness he never had the opportunity to do any more damage to the human race, because he was struck off.

Another young lady received a bad fall when clambering over a hedge in fields near her home. She had a very badly fractured leg. Unfortunately she had to have her leg amputated as there was a fear of gangrene setting in. She was a very plucky young lady and always cheerful, making plans for the future and what she was going to do with her life, and how she would cope with a wheel-chair.

But, suddenly she took a turn for the worse, gangrene had spread. The field where she had fallen was used as grazing for horses. It is a well known fact that infection from such an area is extremely dangerous, this is why she had had the amputation in the first place. The fact that there were no drugs available for the treatment that was needed, plus the poor diet causing some malnutrition, did not help matters at all. That girl fought a losing battle. Her parents were devastated, as she was an only child.

We all felt sad at her loss. It all seemed such a waste of young life.

— — — — —

Now for the lighter side on women's surgical.

As I have already stated, outside the ward the balconies overlooked the yard, and across the meadow on to the hill where some of the German troops were billeted and had a gun emplacement. Every time allied 'planes flew over on their way to France, the Germans who were trigger happy, would be firing "everything" with no chance of hitting "anything".

At night it was not a very comforting thought to know there were bound to be bits of shrapnel dropping all around. This caused us quite a bit of hassle, as the outdoor patients weren't very happy. I always tried to go out there and sit with them at these times until the firing stopped. It can't have been a very pleasant feeling to be bedridden, just lying there waiting to be hit.

These patients were long term and we all got to know each other well. They enjoyed the Nurses' banter and gossip and all the little secrets that young people have. They also enjoyed hearing of all the practical jokes that went on among the staff.

If a certain Male Nurse was on night duty we could be sure there would be many a trick played on us during the night. We just prepared ourselves for the inevitable. For instance, if you had to fetch something from the bathroom at the end of the ward, you'd rush in only to stop dead in your tracks to see someone swinging from the centre-light – a pair of pyjamas stuffed.

Another time you'd go to switch a light on, only to feel not a switch but a cold clammy hand – a rubber glove blown up and all "goo-eey". You just didn't know what you would see or hear next, as no one was safe when he was around.

Enough was enough. We just had to retaliate. We had to give him a dose of his own medicine. But how and what?

After a lot of thought and very careful planning, on a chosen night, when we weren't too busy, it was made known that we had one very sick lady we didn't think would last the night and warned the Male Nurses that they may be called upon to take the corpse down to the mortuary. – No porters and no lifts in those days.

The Night Sister was in on the plan, she helped quite a bit and the other Male Nurse was tipped off as to what would happen. At about 3 a.m. Sister asked the boys to bring in the mortuary stretcher and poles to convey the body down to the mortuary. Everything was made ready for them in the usual way. They carried the 'corpse' down two flights of concrete stairs, occasionally bumping on a stair; then on down the garden path.

It was a beautiful moonlit night. Sister was escorting the case, as was usual. Just before they reached the mortuary door Sister "nudged" the "corpse" and the body sat up, wrapped in a sheet, lifted her arms and yelled (not too loud). Did our victim drop the stretcher and run? No, he just stood there and said "I had a feeling something wasn't quite right"! The poor Nurse who was acting the corpse had endured being bumped down those concrete stairs, she was well bruised, and had been half smothered under the sheets, not daring to breathe too much. The rest of us in the know, were hanging out of the window hoping to see a dramatic finish, and it had all fallen flat! We just couldn't get the better of that man.

When we came on night duty a few days later, day staff were pleased to let us know that they had got our "menace" worried early that morning. Before our joker had finished duty, with the help of some of the outdoor staff, they had hoisted his bike up unto the roof of the balcony and everyone was delighted to watch him hunt high and low for it, until they took pity on him, and put him out of his misery and let him go off home to bed. I must add, he still wasn't cured. We still had to endure his practical jokes.

As mentioned before, on nights we used to have our main meal in two shifts with night staff from other wards. But for tea-time at 4 a.m. each ward had their own arrangements.

If we weren't too busy, this enabled us to, at times, have a little treat as we were just three of us, two Nurses and Sister. Maybe one of us would have been able to purchase a tasty snack of some sort which we would share, before starting on the early morning rush.

One thing we often enjoyed was carrageen pudding, a sort of custard. The carrageen moss, a seaweed, having been gathered at low tide, was vigorously washed then dried in the sun. It was quite a long process. The moss was boiled in milk until it thickened, it didn't have a very pleasant taste, but we soon remedied that by gathering some leaves from an almond tree which was growing down by the mortuary. These leaves were washed and broken up and added to the mixture, it made a deliciously flavoured "almond pudding" when strained. That, washed down with bramble tea, made a lovely snack.

Sometimes we'd collect our odd scraps of bread and make up some bread and milk, leave it to simmer on top of the Aga to thicken, and then fish out most of the husks (the bread was full of them.). As someone once said, "I'm sure they make our bread with the sweepings of the floor, goodness knows what's in it!" No matter. It tasted good and filled a corner. If we were lucky one of us may have had a spoonful of sugar beet syrup to add to the mixture and enhance the flavour.

One night we had a very special treat. During the previous day I had visited my sister and brother-in-law. They had given me some ormers, just three, one for each of us. Ormers are a shell fish gathered at very low tides from under the rocks. They are, and always have been, a great delicacy much sought after by the islanders. The fishermen were always escorted by the Germans and had to part with a percentage of their catches. Maybe that's how my ormers came about, I don't know. There was a fisherman in the family, but I didn't ask anything. One didn't query that sort of thing in those days.

I was so pleased to have something to share with the girls that night. My ormers had been shelled and cleaned, but had not been beaten, which was necessary to tenderize them. So I was out on the stairway, in the early hours of the morning, giving them a good beating with a rolling pin, forgetting that sound echoes up and down the stair well.

Later in the morning a lady patient remarked that the Germans had been playing with their "ack-ack" guns during the night. I was just about to contradict her when I remembered the ormers, so managed to steer the conversation away from guns! Poor patients, if they had known that we staff had had a tea of ormers at 4 a.m., it would have been very hard to face them.

Early mornings were one mad rush when on night duty. We started at 5 a.m., much to the disgust of the patients. It was an enamel bowl of water to each patient who could wash herself sitting up in bed, plus an enamel mug for teeth washing. Then we'd wash those who were unable to help themselves, take round bed-pans and do the backs. Then there was another rush to collect and empty all the bowls, fold towels, straighten lockers, beds etc. and get ready for breakfast. Collecting the bowls of dirty water and dashing to the sluice to empty them was an automatic routine.

"Have you finished with your washing bowl Mrs. .... ? Have you done your teeth?" "Yes thank you Nurse." O.K. One more dash to the sluice, then it would be, "Get the breakfasts done!"

Last bowl emptied, last tooth mug emptied – with a clatter – "Oh, no!" Granny must have left her teeth in the mug. Why, oh why, didn't I check before emptying. I looked, couldn't see <u>anything</u> down the sluice. "Oh, well!" only one thing for it. "Take a deep breath, my girl and think of England! stick your hand and arm down there and 'Hurrah'! I've found Granny's teeth, fine! But are they broken or cracked? A thorough examination whilst washing them under a running tap. Meanwhile my colleague is shouting blue murder.

"What on earth are you doing still mucking about in the sluice while patients are waiting for their breakfast?"

"Sorry, being as quick as I can. Be with you in a minute!"

Wonder of wonders, I couldn't find any damage to the teeth so, I cleaned and cleaned them several times as quickly as possible and then, all smiles, took Granny her teeth in a nice fresh clean mug. "You forgot to put your teeth in ready for your breakfast, Granny, I've given them a clean for you."

"Oh, thank you Nurse, so kind." Did I feel a heel? Oh yes! She was such a sweet old lady. I felt just awful, standing there watching her put her teeth in her mouth. If she had had any idea <u>where</u> they'd been! It doesn't bear thinking about. Thank goodness there were no ill effects.

— — — — —

I pray in the morning as I arise,
   That my duty for the day be well done,
Not for any reward or prize
   But, to feel I have helped someone.

A cheerful "Good-day!" always brings a smile,
   And a kindly act counts a lot.
A simple word, just once in a while
   Nothing to me; but to others a lot.

And so I pray, that throughout the day,
   To help pay a very big debt,
I manage to help other folk on their way
   Their troubles and ills to forget.

B.S.L.

FACING THE CHALLENGES

We had many ups and downs over the years, and experienced so many different cases, with an assortment of complications. We met many folk in all stations of life. So often it would be someone we knew well and it was a pleasure to help get them fit again. But, there were times when we felt so helpless. We were dealing with life and death every day.

Many young people died during that time. This was often due to the lack of right food, also heating and necessary drugs and remedies being unavailable.

Naturally, being such a close-knit community, we felt the loss of folk we knew that much more. For instance, a girl I was at school with and had known most of my life, had undergone a straight-forward appendectomy. Checking that everyone on the ward was O.K. before going off duty one evening, I stopped and had a few words with this girl, who was progressing very favourably. We had a little chat and a laugh and I said, "See you in the morning. Good night everyone!"

Just as I was going out of the door, one of the patients called out, "Nurse, come quickly!" I rushed back to the girl's bedside to find she had collapsed. I screened her off and went for senior help, knowing it would all be in vain. for she had had an embolism. A dreadful shock for everyone, particularly her family who had visited her that afternoon and found her looking so well.

The shocks were hard to take at times.

A married friend, who had been hoping for a family for quite some time, was admitted with a threatened miscarriage five months into her pregnancy. Once again I was just awaiting the Night Staff to finish taking report so that I could go off duty when I realized this friend was in a great deal of pain and discomfort. I went for the Sister who came immediately and between us we did what we could, but the child was aborted. It lived for a few minutes and the Sister, who was a staunch Catholic, asked me to hold the baby while she baptized it, which I found a very moving experience.

It was then my job to tell that friend exactly what had happened. As we both belonged to the same Church I knew she would be strong. She was very grateful to the Sister for her kindly action and was happy that the little one had been blessed.

Another sad occasion I was involved in was on the men's ward, during night duty.

A young lad in his teens had been very ill at home with heart trouble. He was rushed in one night, his condition having worsened. Always very cheerful in spite of being so ill, he won the admiration of all who met him.

In those days, strange as it may seem, no male wore his hair long, but this lad, due I suppose to his having been ill for so long, had not had his hair cut for quite a while. He had beautiful shoulder length dark curly hair, and was a very good-looking lad. He continually made jokes about how good he would look playing his harp and that he would show up all the other angels.

He knew his time was short and was very brave and never complained. Having been with us for a short time, he passed away very peacefully one night. We were so sad that we hadn't been able to do more for him.

Whenever anyone died it was the responsibility of whoever had attended the deceased to check that everything was as it should be in the mortuary, before going off duty. That particular morning after a very busy night, it was my duty to go and do the checking. I was extremely tired and thought I must be imagining things, as the body was still warm.

Common-sense told me he **was** dead, but I **was** very concerned.

On my way back to the ward, I bumped into another Nurse well-known to me. I quickly explained things to her and got her to come back with me to the mortuary. We checked again together and no, it wasn't my imagination, the body was still warm. I reported to Sister, and she in her turn checked and was sure he was dead but couldn't explain the warmth.

Hours later when the deceased's Doctor arrived he went to check the body. (I should have been off duty and in bed by now, but just couldn't rest until I knew the reason for the strange occurrence). We were told that the reason for the unexpected warmth was that during the illness the body had retained so much fluid that rigor mortis took that much longer to set in. The fluid took a time to cool.

One became used to visiting the mortuary, not always a pleasant task. We, one and all, respected the dead and also sympathised with the deceased's relatives. One of our many duties was to take relatives down to see their loved ones. Not very nice for anyone not having experienced such a thing before. Nothing was presented anywhere near today's standard and it was just the stark reality of marble slabs in a row, those occupied discreetly draped in white sheets.

There were many stories about mortuaries and some quite gruesome ones. We got hardened to a lot, but when overtired one's reactions were not quite the same.

Attending one corpse with another Nurse, checking that everything was as it should be, the Nurse accompanying me bent down to retrieve something from the floor when she suddenly jumped up and said to me, "That's _not_ funny, what did you do that for:" Standing the other side of the slab, I said I hadn't done anything. What did she mean? What was wrong? "You hit me," she said, "and it's no joke!" I replied that _she_ must be joking, I hadn't moved at all. I couldn't possibly reach her. Then I saw her white face. She was certain someone had touched her. Thinking there must be somebody else in there besides us we looked about, then realized that the corpse on the next slab had not been placed as it should and an arm had dropped and the Nurse had knocked it as she bent down. We certainly got frights at times. I jokingly said, "It's not everybody who gets a slap on the bottom from a corpse!" We just had to see the funny side of things, otherwise we'd have gone mad. A sense of humour certainly helped keep us sane.

A fine young man who had undergone quite a tricky abdominal operation, was in dire trouble with the German authorities. He had been quite genuinely very ill. The Germans kept checking up on him to see that he was still with us. They were awaiting his discharge to charge him with what they took to be very serious offences.

I do not wish to cause any embarrassment to anyone by stating what he had done, but, he had enabled many an islander to have a decent meal now and then. He knew he was in for very serious punishment from the Germans. We never knew all the facts. Sadly he died very suddenly in the hospital. It's not for me to say how or why. Thankfully he was at rest and was spoken of with much respect for what he had accomplished for his fellow islanders, to the extent of giving his life.

— — — —

There was an elderly Doctor on the Staff who had spent years as a young Army Doctor in the colonies, he was of a very hard school.

He never seemed to have any sympathy or real feeling for his patients, or anyone else for that matter. He was clever and knew his job, but it was his attitude that got to us. He seemed to delight in cleaning up and stitching wounds without any anaesthetic at all and would rave on about when he was abroad he had "Even amputated (to use his expression) a nigger's leg without anaesthetic while he was being held down, and he didn't moan as you are doing for just a few stitches" or whatever.

It made one sick to have to stand by and watch him torture people so unnecessarily. All complaints from the Nursing Staff just made no difference at all. He was such a contrast from the rest of the very caring Doctors.

The saying goes that "every dog has his day". That man had it coming to him. He was admitted for quite minor troubles, which necessitated a little visit to the theatre for tests and examinations. Did I dream it or did I see a "glint" in the eye of every member of the staff who had dealings with him? Yes we had him where we wanted him (not in a malicious way). It was just my luck to be on theatre duty at that time. I kept well in the background when I could. Nurses on his ward reported that they just couldn't do anything right, only to look at him would cause him to moan. I must say the braver ones on duty didn't let him forget the way he spoke to and treated some of his patients. The Male nurses had the time of their lives when attending to him.

When he was on the operating table, the surgeon whom he had delegated to look after him, being a man of great patience and kindness, took all sorts of abuse from the old chap during the examinations. Seeing he couldn't in any way ruffle the surgeon, he then started on Matron, who was assisting. He kept complaining he was thirsty and he was very uncomfortable, to say nothing of the terrible pain he was suffering.

Matron motioned me to her side and sent me off on a mission. When I returned she said, "Nurse, give some of those to the Doctor, he's being such a baby, maybe if he sucks on those he'll forget about what's going on and keep quiet while we sort him out." I could see she was having a good laugh behind her mask. I did feel a fool. There was I feeding the "old boy" on sugar lumps, a very precious few which Matron had saved for some reason of her own.

I had been dispatched to her sitting room to search for these sugar lumps in her cupboard. There were only a few in a small screw-top jar. At least our patient did shut up for a bit. When he had been returned to the ward, we just collapsed laughing.

Poor man he was <u>so</u> difficult to get on with. Many's the time he'd argue with the younger Doctors. He was living in the past and his language often turned the air blue. I can't remember if he learnt anything during his stay as a patient. I think not. He was too old to change his ways.

It was he who reported me to Matron once. At that time I was working on the Children's Ward. I'd not heard him come in, so on entering the little kitchen at the end of the ward I was amazed to find him behind the door of the food cupboard. I had surprised him and he turned towards me with a plate in his hand on which was a small knob of butter, the kids' ration for the day. I asked him what he thought he was doing, to which he replied, "Is this Guernsey butter?" and stuck his finger in it and licked his finger. I was so furious, I didn't think what I was doing. I snatched the plate from his hand and smacked his face saying, "Just keep your fingers out of the children's butter ration." He just stormed out and, yes, half an hour later, I was "on the carpet". Matron wanted to see me in her sitting room. Oh, dear!

I was met with her sternest glare. "What's this I hear about your behaviour toward a Doctor, Nurse, explain yourself." This I did feeling dreadful, knowing I should never have done such a thing, expecting a real telling off at least.

When I plucked up enough courage to look up and face Matron fair and square, it was to see her laughing. I was so surprised. "Good for you, Nurse. I would have done the same!"

But then, of course, she did remind me that that was really not the way to behave toward a Doctor. Point taken.

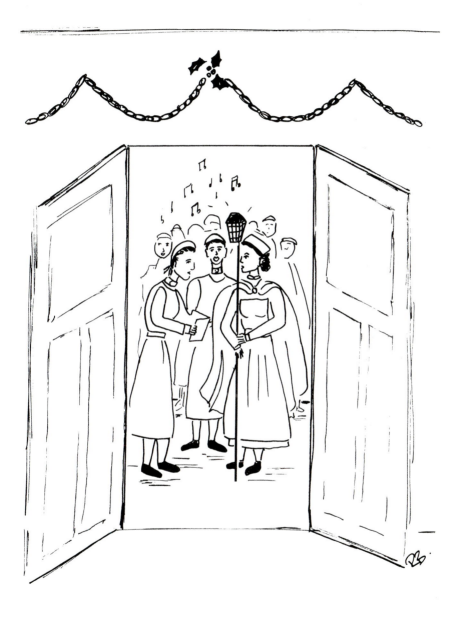

Christmas Morning Carols

CHRISTMAS CAROLS

As Christmas approached, patients who were well enough were encouraged to help make paper flowers and other decorations with whatever material was available.

Each ward would plan and work on their own theme with as much secrecy as possible. There was stiff competition between the wards. Some of us would stay and help out after finishing duty, determined that our ward would be the best. A lot of our off-duty time was spent in the "Rec" too, around the piano, practising carols. It was a very busy time for everyone. Christmas, as always, came around much too soon.

I'm writing about the <u>first</u> Christmas of the occupation, before too many things became too short.

One rule at this time was that Christmas Day was the Patients' Day and none of the Nursing Staff had any off-duty. We did have our Christmas dinner, all Nursing Staff from Matrons down to latest probationer, not forgetting our Resident Doctor.

Christmas morning, between 7 and 7.30 a.m., as many of the nursing staff as possible met in the "Recreation Room". that is Nurses from all the wards on all floors, Medical, Maternity and Surgical, leaving just a skeleton staff on duty.

When we were all gathered together, all spruced up in fresh uniforms, with red-lined capes and lanterns held high, we set off carol singing. Walking first right through the kitchens, where they were all very busy preparing the Christmas Fayre and Cook was crying into our porridge, because we all "looked so lovely and sounded so nice"!

We'd then wend our way up the first flight of stairs, singing all the way, voices echoing up through the great stairways. Into the women's surgical ward, right down and through the open double doors on to the landing, through the doors of the men's surgical.

I must say there was many a moist eye among the patients and those who were able, joined in with the carol singing. Out of the far end of men's ward and up the next flight of stairs and into the medical men's and then women's wards, across the landing and we were in the maternity ward, where we always sang "Away in a manger". There was always that extra special feeling on that ward on Christmas Day.

Onward and up another flight of stairs, along the corridor where the Matrons' bedrooms were, also the Resident Doctor's room, still singing and shouting "Merry Christmas" as we passed each individual door. The Doctor stuck his head out of his bathroom door and hailed us with his face fully lathered, much to our amusement.

When we got to the top of the building, we all gathered around a large window which overlooked the buildings on the hillside where some troops were living. After having the window up as high as possible, we all took a deep breath and sang as loud as we could, "Land of Hope and Glory" and "God save the King", our National Anthem – both of which were "*verboten*" by the Kommandant – Gosh! We did feel good after that. Just the thought of defying orders gave us a boost. Then amidst a lot of chattering and laughing it was back downstairs to get to work!

What an atmosphere right through the hospital, everyone was happy (we almost forgot we were occupied).

The night staff had made all the beds for us, and many other little duties, thus enabling the day staff to spend more time with the patients, entertaining them as best we could, having a chat while they displayed gifts they'd received.

The doors connecting the male and female surgical were left open so the staff were able to mix freely among all patients on that floor. Only the essential dressings and medications were done that day, just the bare necessities.

During the latter part of the morning all the Doctors came round to visit their patients and wish them a "Happy Christmas". Some of them came armed with mistletoe, which all added to the fun. The patients enjoyed watching the Sisters and Nurses being chased around the wards by Doctors and Male Nurses.

When the ward dinners were finished, and the patients encouraged to have a rest before their visitors arrived, it was time for the staff dinner.

Three large tables were set in our dining room. One across the top for the Resident doctor, Matrons and Sisters. The two long tables at the sides were for the rest of us. It was traditional that all the Nursing Staff, night staff included, had Christmas Dinner together.

What of the patients you ask? Well, the domestics were left in charge and would call if circumstances required it. (The Sisters did take it in turns to take a "shifty" now and then.) I must say the domestics were very good.

This first Christmas was a very good traditional one, as the rations and cut-backs had not yet been too severe. And thanks to our wonderful Caterer, who must have planned well ahead, we had a very good dinner. So did the patients.

We had the usual Bran Tub. Each member of the staff had donated a gift up to a certain agreed price. The Doctor had the job of handing out the gifts after the meal.

With "tummies" full and feeling very pleased with ourselves, it was back on the wards, to be greeted by the domestics who'd held the "fort".

"Everything is alright, Nurse, no one has had any trouble. And we've done the bed-pan round for you, and the sluice is all clean and tidy." "Bless them." So many times have Nurses' ears burned during everyday work. Nurses always made Domestics' life hell. This was Christmas with a capital "C". What Christmas is all about.

After visitors and tea, it was a lick and promise all around and a general freshen up and patients were made comfortable. Then it was more singing and bits of fun. The poor old ward piano was truly "pounded".

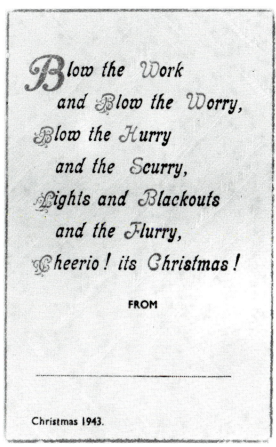

Christmas Card

All the patients just loved to see the Nurses make fools of themselves, and we could generally find some little joke to crack about patients in the various little skits we would enact for them, all in good fun of course.

After supper, a Male Nurse would stand between the two wards and play his piano-accordion and with dimmed lights throughout the wards, all the staff would dance through from one ward to the other.

When it was time for the Day staff to go off duty, they'd stay a little later to have a bit of fun with the Night Staff, before helping to tuck up the very tired patients for the night. Tired but happy.

I've completely forgotten to mention "Charlie". How could I be so remiss.

"Charlie" was very popular with staff and patients. One of the Male Nurses was quite a clever ventriloquist. "Charlie" was his doll. Everyone enjoyed this act, which often appeared throughout the hospital and recreation room. He also appeared in some of the Amateur Dramatic Society performances in the Little Theatre in town.

Boxing Day was the Domestics' Day. They had stood in for us Christmas Day, so it was our chance to show how much we appreciated their good work.

They all had their Christmas Dinner that day together, we did their work for them, the ward dishes and cleaning up.

The Male Nurses volunteered to wait on them all, so that they could relax and enjoy themselves. From all the laughter we could hear from their dining-room, I'm sure a good time was had by all!

We always put on a Nativity Play for the patients. A group of Nurses would enact the Nativity during the Christmas period to each ward in turn. It was always a moving thing to do on Maternity Ward, always very special. Everyone enjoyed it and would join in with the carols.

As the years went by the Christmases became more lean, but no less joyful. And each Christmas we would say, "Next year we'll have a proper Christmas, everything will be over this time next year!"

THE OCCUPYING FORCES

The German troops, too, celebrated Christmas. We could hear those billeted near us singing carols in harmony, which sounded lovely. They, like ourselves, no doubt thinking of their loved ones so many miles away.

Quite frequently they would sing whilst out on route marches. The chorus of "The Happy Wanderer, Fal-de-ree, Fal-de-ra ... !" echoing through the surrounding country lanes. The outside patients enjoyed the singing. Sadly, there came the time when those men no longer sang or even felt like singing. They realized things were not going their way.

We were very fortunate that in the first place we had a very understanding Kommandant, who treated us as best he could, and generally things weren't too bad. It was the silly, stupid orders that got us down. Mind you, many of the islanders saw the funny side of these orders and as long as we humoured Jerry we were alright.

But, unfortunately, all good things come to an end, and Hitler discovered that the island was being treated too leniently for his liking, so, our Kommandant was replaced; apparently he had British family connections.

We were sorry when he left, even more sorry when we found that his replacement was a real Nazi. This happened toward the end of the occupation. Everyone was very upset when we heard later, that the young Kommandant who had been kind to us, had been taken back to Germany, thoroughly reprimanded, and eventually shot for not carrying out his duties as he should have done.

Things in general became worse and worse. Petrol was very scarce and what little there was was allocated only for the most essential journeys. Doctors had to resort to cycles for most of their calls, keeping what small amounts of petrol they had for emergency use.

It was no joke cycling round the island with so many hills and on such meagre rations. More and more people were admitted for treatment which would have normally been dealt with at home, as the Doctors just couldn't cope with distant calls.

The St. John Ambulance had adapted to the use of gas on an ambulance for a time. They later resorted to using a horse-drawn vehicle which looked something like an old covered wagon. It was painted white with the St. John logo in black, with black finishings and was drawn by two black horses. It looked very smart and, much to the amusement of the Ambulance lads, some of the Germans thought it only right and proper to salute as it went by, as they thought it was a hearse.

This vehicle was not much use in an emergency; they kept the motorized ambulance for that. The horse-drawn one was O.K. for taking patients home or picking up non-emergency cases. The hospital wards co-operated with discharges, and tried to get together folk from more or less the same areas.

As it was such a slow moving vehicle it was not much use for maternity cases; without anything else, our road repairs having been neglected and with the very heavy German traffic, there were many bumps and holes in the roads which would not have been very comfortable for the Mums-to-be. So it was arranged that expectant Mums be admitted at least a week before baby was due, which saved a lot of worry all round.

It was quite a common sight to see a bunch of heavily pregnant women taking their constitutional through the lanes surrounding the hospital, amid much chatter and laughter, all very friendly.

We had our personal clothing, as well as our uniforms, laundered every week by the hospital laundry. In the course of time our clothing, mufti and uniform, wore out and became very shabby. Towards the end of the occupation several of the staff were dressed in a variety of coloured uniforms. Stockings and shoes were also hard to get hold of, and if one wasn't careful most of one's belongings "grew legs". Small items like fountain pens and scissors, besides shoes and odd bits of clothing, all "walked".

The laundry staff worked hard and did the best they could with whatever was available. But there came a time when whites were far from white; bed linen, table linen, gowns, aprons, all became a horrible grey, also a lot of linen was not ironed. When the linen was washed in awful smelly soaps, the smell seemed to linger on the sheets.

A lot of the laundry machines had to be left out of use owing to lack of power. The heating for the water was kept going by the use of tar. The boiler that had been adapted was fed from the top with buckets of tar poured in, which ran down through piping and sprayed on to the fire bars. That was for the laundry.

The water for the main part of the hospital, i.e. for patients' wards, theatre, kitchens etc., was heated by a different boiler which was fed with whatever fuel was available at the time. Mains electricity was rationed, but there was a stand-by generator for theatre and labour ward for use in emergency.

— — — — —

Ward work was unceasing with a regular run of admissions and discharges. The sick had to be cared for. I can honestly say that they all received all the care and treatment needed with what drugs we had available.

Our actual duties didn't change at all, the routine and the discipline was kept up throughout all the hazards we had to cope with.

Washings, feedings, treatments, temperatures taken, backs rubbed, and without fail the Blanket-Baths. The patient was stripped from top to toe while lying between two blankets and then every bit of the patient was washed. Can you imagine the moans and groans we had to put up with, particularly on the men's ward. Mind you, we gave as good as we got and too much cheek and we'd find a job for them to help out with.

Whilst preparing the next victim we'd give the last one the job of changing the pillow slips, a simple enough job, but that's where we got caught out with one chap. It was usual practice to strip the beds of discharged patients, mattresses and all, and then wash down the bed before making it up for the next patient. On clearing this particular patient's bedding, the pillow slips had to be removed for the laundry and clean ones replaced. Nurse took off the dirty pillow slip for the laundry, only to find another one under it, and another and another. She finished up with about six pillow slips from his pillow. That patient had put the clean one on top of the dirty one every time!

Giving out medicines was another task. The one medicine I disliked handing to the patient was "castor oil", it just turned my stomach to see the stuff. The majority of the patients hated taking it too and there was I, all smiles and encouraging words, trying to "help the medicine go down", feeling queasy as I watched the patient drink it up to the very last drop.

There came a time when everyone was becoming despondent, longing for something to happen, all waiting and waiting. For _what_? We'd seen and heard wave upon wave of R.A.F. 'planes flying over to France and hoped and prayed that things would soon change for the better. At times we could hear the rumbling of the bombing and see flashes and glares of the explosions over France's skyline. The theme was always: "It just can't go on for much longer. It will soon be over!" Wishful thinking!

We all hoped we'd be freed before another winter and having to face the threat of starvation. The rations at that time hardly kept body and soul together. With these things in mind, just imagine our excitement when we heard that a Red Cross Ship was on its way. But seeing the announcement in the "Press" put in by the Germans, made one wonder, was it just another rumour? We had got to the stage of not knowing who or what to believe.

A few days later it was confirmed. The Red Cross Ship was "en route" for the Channel Islands. As you can imagine the conversation from then on was unquestionably "Food Parcels". When will they be here? What will they contain? We each had our yearnings for various things. Types of food we hadn't seen for years. I even bargained with one young Nurse that if my parcel contained some chocolate and her's didn't but had some soap, we'd do a 'swop'. I just longed for a good bath with lovely lathery soap, instead of gritting muck, to say nothing of a sweet scent.

As it turned out no swop was necessary, we received both chocolate and soap in our parcels.

I was working on the women's surgical at the time, and I promised our two long stay patients out on the balcony, that if I received my parcel before they received theirs, I would open mine with them.

Well, the great day came, and on 27th December 1944 the "Vega" docked and on the 31st the parcels were distributed, one for each civilian, with special ones for babies.

What rejoicing there was! What excitement! And many, many tears of happiness. Smiling faces everywhere.

These parcels were Canadian, the first we received. Later we had some from New Zealand as well. We can never thank them enough.

I kept my promise. I received my parcel as I went off duty, then made a dash up the fire escape to my two friends on the balcony, drew up a chair between their beds, hoping I wouldn't get caught out by Sister. Come to think of it she most likely would have turned a blind eye, as I was off duty, though still in uniform.

The excitement was intense. We were so thrilled to see food we had been dreaming of, and talking about, for so long. The patients had to wait until their relations brought their parcels in on the next visiting day.

The contents of the box included:

Biscuits, a type of ship's biscuit, large, round, very hard and thick, they were ideal either soaked in milk, or just nibbled with butter or jam on. Very welcome.

Tinned milk, condensed, flavoured with coffee, which made instant coffee with hot water.

A whole pound of butter (tin).

Tinned meats, tinned fruit.

A block of chocolate in a tin.

Cheese, dried fruit, powdered milk and

TEA, which at that time was £16 a pound on the Black Market.

Also a large tablet of toilet soap.

— — — —

Strange how little things stick in one's mind. I well remember how, when we collected the flowers from the patients, we loved to see the red nerines that were sometimes brought in. The scent of these was similar to the smell of chocolate and everyone would have a jolly good sniff and dream; such silly things meant so much.

Back to the parcels. Many islanders, quite understandably, made themselves ill through eating too much rich food too quickly, even though everyone was warned by Doctors to go easy on all the goodies. Our tummies were not used to so much richness.

As I've already said there was many a tear shed over the wonderful gifts of food. We will never forget the kindness and generosity of the Canadians and New Zealanders who gave so much. Also the Red Cross Society and St. John Ambulance Association and, last but not least, the Captain and Crew of the ship the "Vega" who visited us more than once with so many essentials without which we most surely would have starved.

At last we felt we had not been forgotten, which helped us to bravely face up to "whatever!". But we couldn't help but wonder what the "whatever" would be, or how much longer we'd have to wait.

Receiving the parcels solved many problems, not the least finding some sort of snack for the Resident Doctor who, when doing his round every night, looked forward to whatever night staff could find for him. Many times it was just a hot drink, but what he really enjoyed was what he called a "heel" (a crust of bread). However, come to think of it, I don't suppose he did too badly as by the time he'd called on each ward and had a 'snack' on most, it must have helped fill up more than a corner. He certainly appreciated everyone's efforts.

Work on the wards went on. Patients took a long time to heal and pick up enough strength to see them home again. Many of the staff were suffering from dysentery, amongst other things. Care had to be taken if one received a scratch or cut; if ignored it would soon become septic.

Night duty was a strain. We found it difficult to keep alert and devised all sorts of things to help pass the time, but there's only so much one can do when sitting in the dark.

One elderly Sister, who was really very sweet, would find it very difficult. We'd desperately try and find something of interest to discuss, or talk about, but she'd often "nod" off, much to the amusement of us youngsters. Sometimes she'd say "I'm just going down to Matron's sitting-room, there's something I have to attend to for her. If you need me you'll know where I am, Nurse." "Yes, of course, Sister."

Then we'd have a little "giggle", knowing that if she was needed, it would be a toss up as to <u>who</u> would go down to fetch her, as it would be rather embarrassing to have to awaken her from her deep sleep, stretched out on Matron's settee. We did feel sorry for her deep down, she wasn't as young as us, we could fight that much harder. It must have been a great trial for her to keep going.

There was one experience on night duty that none of us enjoyed. It seemed to happen towards the end of a long stint on nights. That was "night nurses' paralysis" really frightening. Suddenly you'd become conscious of needing to move from your chair, either to do a round, or answer a call from the ward, or even just to answer a colleague next to you, only to find you couldn't move or speak; it would only last a matter of seconds but felt like hours. You would try to call your colleague to give you a shove, but no sound would come. You'd be conscious of all that was happening around you, but unable to do a thing about it. If you were fortunate enough to have someone with you who had experienced this, it was a great help, as they would recognise what was happening and thankfully help you out by giving you a good jolt.

GHOSTS

As I have previously mentioned, the hospital building is very old. Known originally as "The Country Hospital"; now the Câtel Hospital, during war years "The Emergency Hospital".

Being so old, there were typically many stories of ghosts and lots of horrible happenings over the years. Some of the rooms at the top of the building were supposedly haunted; one by a girl who had hanged herself, and there were numerous accounts of different occurrences.

During conversation at the breakfast table one morning, together with the night staff of the other wards, the subject of ghosts arose, and we discussed various tales that we'd heard. Eventually we plucked up the courage to get up from the table and go off to our well-earned rest. All too soon the alarm would wake us for another night's work.

Back on duty that night, someone brought up the subject of ghosts yet again. Night staff on women's surgical always went over to the men's surgical to have their main meal in the duty room there, and we were always joined by the staff from the Maternity Floor.

The duty room, where we ate, had very large windows which overlooked the lodge gate and on to the main driveway. Immediately below our windows were the windows of the Medical Staff duty room, where they partook of their main meal on nights.

During dinner, again the same subject came up. We could hear our colleagues below laughing and chatting over their meal. Always ready for a laugh and to cheer ourselves up a bit, we thought we'd invent a ghost. There was always a lot of rivalry between the wards, one lot always trying to out-do the other.

It was a beautiful moonlit night, so having tied a long piece of string on to a pair of scissors, we switched our light off so as to move the black-out, opened the window wide and lowered the scissors level with the window below. A gentle swaying movement produced a clear "tap" on their window, but they were chatting too much and didn't hear it. We waited for a lull in the conversation and gave three distinctive "taps". Dead silence; then, "What was that?" Giggles from our end. That was a start. Next morning in the dining room we met our colleagues for breakfast and discussed many things, then we were told of the weird tappings that they had heard at about 1 a.m. "No! we hadn't heard any tappings!" We did point out, however, that they were on the ground floor and with curfew it couldn't have been anyone in the driveway. Or could it?

Next night at precisely the same time, we delivered three more taps. At breakfast we had the full story of how it had happened again, and that the male nurse even went outside to see who was there, but, he didn't see anyone or anything. All this, of course, we knew. He didn't dream of looking up to where we were huddled together watching him, and we could tell he was pretty scared to be out there on his own.

We were really rotten to them, and kept up the tappings for about a week, just "three" taps at precisely the same time every night. They even went out two together and stood in the doorway waiting to catch the culprit, and just couldn't understand how the taps continued when no one was in sight.

Came the time when our night duty was due to end, we would soon be going over to 'days', so we agreed to put them out of their misery, and let them discover how the tappings were delivered by hanging out of our window so that we could be seen. We certainly got a fair amount of whispered abuse that night, and became the topic of conversation in the dining-room for a while.

It all sounds so childish now, but we had to do something to keep our spirits up, and it was all in good fun. They'd find a way of getting back at us, you may be sure.

One thing I must point out. No way were the patients neglected. Our meals were taken in shifts. There was <u>always</u> staff on the wards. Our meal times were our own time.

REAL HUNGER

There came a time when everybody and every living thing became more and more hungry. It was almost impossible to keep what little bits of food we did have in our digs safe from mice.

The majority of cats had disappeared at an alarming rate. The Germans were hungry too and were eating them – so the mice were multiplying and like every living creature at the time, they too were hungry and became very tame. Being billeted in an old cottage which was attached to a large barn didn't help matters.

I was lucky enough to have acquired a couple of mouse traps, the old wooden ones with a strong spring, and as we were infested with mice I'd make sure to set the traps, no need for bait as such. 'The girls in the next room were scared of mice, but wouldn't do anything to catch them.

I'd be awakened by the "snap" of the traps, get out of bed, take the dead mouse out, reset the trap and get back to bed, checking first that the mice hadn't had the cheek to get in there before me! The traps would go off three or four times a night. More than once I awoke to find a mouse had disturbed me by running over my pillow and over the bed. So we had to protect everything as best we could, and make sure that all that could shut was shut.

I always slept with my hockey-stick on hand, alongside my low divan bed, and sometimes used the stick to try and "whack" the little beggars, but that wasn't very successful, which was just as well, imagine the mess if I had succeeded!

— — — — —

There were several German soldiers billeted nearby. They had to pass literally under my window when going up the lane past the cottage.

One warm, clear night, I was in bed and was disturbed by some scrabbling noises outside my window, which was open. Turning toward the window, I could distinguish two hands on the sill. Quietly and carefully lifting my hockey-stick, I took aim and hit the hands, "one" and "two". There was a shout and a lot of muttering, then footsteps running up the lane. Bet he didn't go climbing up windows again in a hurry. It was a German soldier. My window was set fairly low to the road and there was a very small window below which could be used as a step.

Another evening the Nurse from across the landing was sitting on the end of my bed, we were chatting, sitting in the dark. We could hear some soldiers out in the lane, but took no notice at first, because as I have said before, the troops were pretty well behaved. Once again there was scrambling outside. We were both drinking our evening milk ration. As soon as a face appeared it received most of the milk, and again, there was quite a bit of cursing and off they went.

The Germans were becoming disheartened and feeling the lack of food. How different their attitude toward the islanders was now. But we didn't forget how they acted when first they were here in our island. Although we had no idea <u>what</u> we'd have to face in the near future, one thing was certain in our minds:

"Right <u>would</u> win!" With this in mind we could, and we would, keep right on to the end.

There were very few cats and dogs left on the island. All pets had to be kept indoors, otherwise they too were taken to feed the troops. Folk who had kept and bred rabbits and chickens for their own table over the years, had to bring them all inside the house for safe-keeping. The Germans were so hungry they would steal anything. They were often seen gathering stinging nettles, and anything else they could "pinch" from fields and gardens, to make soup with. Nothing was safe.

We guarded our Red Cross Parcels and had to make sure they were safely hidden. Theft was rife. Houses were broken into and people threatened as Germans hunted for food. They were unable to get their supplies. Nothing at all could come through from France. Our parcels saved us.

The thing I enjoyed most at the end of the day's work (having been going to bed with that "sinking" feeling for so long) was the ship's biscuits, large, thick and hard as rocks. It was lovely to get into bed, to keep warm, and sit there for ages just nibbling at a biscuit, making it last as long as possible and perhaps go mad and have <u>one</u> square of chocolate with it. Or, soak the biscuit in milk when it would swell up to a tremendous size, but it didn't take so long to eat that way.

We didn't know when, or even if, we would receive any more food parcels, so, I tried to eke out what I had. Some of us would share a tin of food, rather than open two at once, and so enjoyed meals together. We had to be careful with such luxuries after such a poor diet. And what a delight to have a real cup of tea. No more of that bramble tea, thank you.

Most of the children on the island had never tasted, or even seen, such foods. They had never tasted chocolate.

What a relief for mothers who had been struggling to satisfy a growing family all these years, often doing without herself so as to feed her children. It must have been a very hard thing to say to your child, "No, you cannot have any more". The parcels were so thankfully received.

That first parcel saved us from actual starvation. Soon after receiving it, the island ran out of flour (such as it had been). We had no bread at all for three weeks.

Families were on very scanty meals, often just one meal a day consisting of maybe, if they still had some, a biscuit and perhaps a little soup of vegetables, skins and all, just chopped up or minced, then boiled. Folk would go to bed to try and keep warm. There was no lighting and no heating. Nothing to entertain, no comforts. We just waited to see what would happen next.

Then, thankfully, the Red Cross Ship, the "Vega", called again with New Zealand parcels and other supplies and, what we'd all been longing for, Flour.

A couple of days later, I saw something that I have never forgotten. When coming off duty I had to pass the kitchens. Just outside was a large store cupboard and standing in the centre with shelves all around her, was our Assistant Caterer, a very sweet motherly soul. There she was standing gazing all around her. I doubt if she could see 'what' she was looking at, as the tears were flowing fast. I stopped to ask if she was alright.

"Oh, yes Nurse; I'm O.K., just look at all this lovely bread!" I had to agree with her. It was a wonderful sight, and I'm not ashamed to say that my tears joined hers.

The wooden shelves were laden with huge pure white "tommy-loaves", row upon row of them. So white, such beautiful golden brown crusts. What a marvellous sight! Bread, glorious bread! That bread was like cake to us. We had been supplied with the very best, the first quality flour.

Guernsey, the isle of plenty,
Has changed these last four years.
No one thought it would empty
And bring forth those hunger tears.

Three weeks we've been without bread
The main stay of our men.
Three weeks of doubt and query –
Will the Red Cross send again?

After such long weeks of waiting
A ship is seen at last.
Each member of the island
Sends a prayer from his heart.

We pray they've sent us flour,
We pray for bread once more,
Was the cry of many people
From Guernsey's sunny shore.

The seventh day of March, folk,
Is one to remember for aye,
When all received a real white loaf,
The answer to many a prayer.

I hope that all have said "Thank you"
To the One who never forgets
And although things looked dark and dreary
Remember, He feeds you yet.

B.S.L.

THE LOCAL "PRESS"

The local "Press" was controlled by the Germans and was fondly called the "Tuppenny Liar". There was very little of general news in it, but plenty of propaganda and orders, orders, and yet more orders. Islanders mustn't do this and they mustn't do that. More restrictions as the Germans were getting very worried. They were laying many more mines around the island, some on private properties.

We were all on edge, afraid that the Germans would panic and that there would be drastic results. They continued to tighten up in every way they could. People felt that nothing was their own any more.

All the stupid rules and regulations were to keep the Guernseyman well and truly under the "Jack-Boot". Any wonder that we were becoming more and more disillusioned.

But suddenly there would be a little ray of sunshine, somebody would have managed to "pick up" a bit of good news. Things were moving on the continent. "Shouldn't be long now!" How many times did we hear that phrase. Every little snippet of news was passed on and well digested.

There were very few 'phones in use, so many lines had been taken over by the Germans and then so many telephone receivers were in use by islanders for other more important things, as receivers for the "crystal sets".

I remember one chap, when passing on some B.B.C. news, said he had accidentally linked up to a German gun emplacement near his home. He got the shock of his life when he heard German voices talking excitedly about the B.B.C. It was a long while before he thought of trying to pick up the B.B.C. again.

Although things seemed to be coming to the end, one couldn't be sure how the Germans might react. It would have been very foolish to get into serious trouble just at that time.

Every day excitement seemed to mount. Some of the troops appeared to have given up, not the Officers, but the ordinary soldiers – they knew they hadn't a hope and were only too pleased to know that the end was in sight. They too had homes and relatives that they were longing to see again. They had had more than enough of war. They were very hungry, weak and tired.

On 6th May (Sunday) we heard on the 6 p.m. news bulletin that Churchill was to make an announcement within the next couple of days, declaring the end of hostilities.

Everyone was on "pins", crystal sets were in continuous use. The men of the family took it in turns to listen in. Radios appeared from their hiding places. Those hours, full of anticipation, were so drawn out. We were longing and hoping for "good news".

One family I know of were asked by some soldiers if they would allow them to listen to the radio, which these folk did, knowing they were decent men who were fed up with everything. Eventually, the speech we'd all been waiting for, was broadcast. Those young Germans jumped for joy. "Hitler Kaput"! they cheered, throwing their hats in the air.

At this time the Germans were still trying to work as if nothing had happened and on the morning of the 8th May some were still laying mines. Then – Rumour was rife once more – "The Germans won't surrender!"

Many islanders congregated near the Harbour and along the front, all looking for the sight of British ships that we knew were in the Channel. Near the Salerie corner was a pre-war radio shop and to the delight of us all, the owner fitted up loud-speakers outside. He must have had all his equipment well and truly hidden over the years.

So many islanders gathered outside that shop, myself included. Most of our off-duty time was spent gathering what news we could to take back to the hospital, trying to keep all in touch with the latest.

The whole time we were waiting outside that shop, two Germans with rowdy motor-cycles, rode up and down making as much noise as possible. Some officers appeared, curious as to what was going on. Everyone just ignored them. I had the impression that they too wanted to hear what Churchill had to say.

What excitement. I think it was about 3 p.m. when the voice of Churchill was heard. There was such cheering, laughter and tears when those, never to be forgotten, words of his came over.

"And our dear Channel Islands shall be liberated at "such and such a time."!" The cheers were so tremendous that many of us missed the full message, but we'd heard enough. Never had the sun shone so brightly. Never had there been such a joyous day. British Flags appeared as if by magic. That was on the 8th May 1945.

On the 9th the first party of British troops landed. (On the 8th six British had landed to prepare for engineers to clear the way for the 3,000 British troops.) What a welcome sight of British Ships and R.A.F. 'planes. What sighs of relief, and smiles and tears of islanders and liberators.

British tanks and lorries were driven off the huge landing craft that just managed to enter the Old Harbour (opposite Woolworths). Actually they couldn't come right in, they dropped the ramp through the entrance and the vehicles drove across the Old Harbour bed and up the slipway.

How we cheered the British Tommies in khaki (we were sick of the horrid grey-green uniforms). The "Jack Tars", all spick and span, R.A.F. men as smart as ever, all looking so clean and fresh.

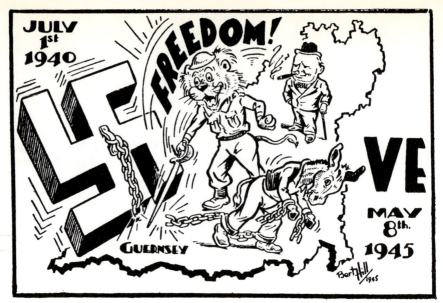

All Rights Reserved—Guernsey Star & Gazette Co., Ltd.

Liberation Card

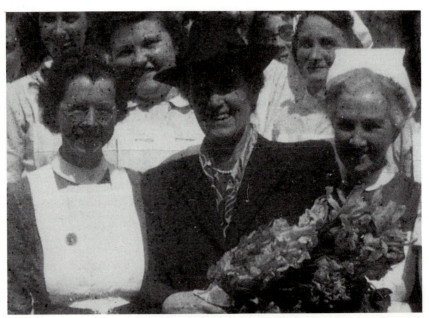

Matron at retirement, with two sisters

So many times I have been asked: "What did it feel like to be liberated?"

After nearly fifty years I still get such a surge of very deep feelings that no words can ever express. Only those who went through the experience can understand, and I doubt if any of them can truly explain.

The British must have found us such a shabby looking lot. Over the years we had been so used to making do and mending and had no fashion conscience at all. Those men must have felt they had gone back in time when they saw our styles and fashions.

What a splendid sight H.M. ships riding at anchor out in the roadsteads were, with smaller vessels and tenders ploughing back and forth. Much activity wherever one looked.

British troops and vehicles were everywhere. Oh, what a splendid sight it was! Not a German at large. The "Brits" were controlling them in a very orderly fashion. Work parties were clearing mines etc. German officers were being ferried off the island, out to H.M. Ships to be transported to the U.K. as prisoners of war.

I'm afraid we didn't have much sympathy for them as we watched them boarding the tenders. Many of them were laden with "spoils", all manner of items they had amassed during their stay. Maybe legally purchased, maybe not. The Tommies were wise to them and many were made to leave these goods behind. (I wonder what happened to all those goods left on the slipway?)

One satisfying sight for us, was to see the Nazi Kommandant publicly stripped of his decorations and marched down to the boat. He had not had the decency to face the British Liberation forces aboard the H.M.S. Bulldog in the first instance. He had had the audacity to send one of his junior officers to sign the treaty.

Needless to say the British weren't putting up with that nonsense and the young officer was quickly sent back "with a flea in his ear". And so there had been a delay in signing the "treaty" until the Kommandant was forced to admit to his error and agree to board the H.M.S. Bulldog and do the necessary.

— — — —

And, what of the hospital during those days? Yes, we were still working and looking after our patients. They were all longing to be up and about to join in all the celebrations, and for the off-duty staff to return to the ward and fill them in with all the latest news of what was happening in the town.

The R.A.F., bless them, did not forget the hospital and at the time of their arrival they flew in low over the hospital, circled round and round dipping their wings. They flew so low that we could clearly see the crews waving and smiling. We responded by waving sheets and bedpans and bottles, anything at hand as they went by. The patients on the balconies had a grandstand view; their very own "fly past".

Something different was happening every day, the excitement was so great, AND NO CURFEW, anyone could stay out all night if they wished, and we were once more driving on the left of the road: Wonder of wonders! We just couldn't take it all in. Everyone was so happy!

— — — —

There's one particular afternoon that stands out vividly in my mind. It was one of the first days of liberation.

I was on the landing between A and B surgical wards, with a colleague. We heard quite a bit of chatting and somebody coming up the stairs at quite a rate. We just had to wait and see who it was (Yes, nosey!). Much to our surprise it was two young sailors, grinning from ear to ear.

"Hello. We wondered if we could visit some of the patients as they must feel they are missing out on such a lot."

We nurses didn't bother about getting permission, we just opened B ward door wide (men's surgical) and ushered them in. We announced to the men "You've got some very special visitors, lads, just look who's here. The Navy's in!"

I've always regretted that I did not find out the names of those boys or the name of the ship they were serving on. Those two lads brought so much joy to everyone. There were patients of varying ages, one or two men who had served in the 1914-18 war. They were all so overwhelmed at the kindness and thoughtfulness of those two Able Seamen. Tears were streaming down the faces of the men, they just couldn't speak at first.

Once they had got over the shock, they were firing questions all the time. Those sailors shook the hand of every one of those patients and wished them well.

We two nurses suddenly came down to earth and one dashed off to notify Matron as to what was going on, while the other rushed across to Women's Ward to give the good news and make sure everything was in order for The Visitors – V.I.P's and make no mistake about it.

The patients who were having bed-baths were very quickly made respectable and everything tidied up. What excitement everywhere. We also notified all the other wards and made sure no one would be left out. It was difficult to keep the boys more or less on the go so that all the patients met them. I'm sure that everyone involved still remembers that afternoon.

One ward the boys visited gave a rousing rendering of "Rule Britannia", much to their embarrassment, but they took it all in good part.

With permission, that visit was the first of many. They spent a lot of their spare time with the patients.

As I've already stated, I wish I had kept a record of those men. I wonder if they realized what delight and joy they brought to that hospital.

Everything was happening so quickly. We had suddenly found ourselves in a very different world. The whole island was changing rapidly.

Goods were once more appearing in the shops. Shops that had been closed and shuttered up for most of the occupation were freshened up and items which we hadn't seen the likes of for years were displayed once again. Some goods and labels and trade marks we hadn't seen before. All was so new to us.

English papers were read over and over and illustrations studied; pictures of the King and Queen and other well known people. There was so much to catch up on.

New styles were shown. Yes, we were taking notice of fashion again. And a vast array of Utility goods. We received extra coupons, also vouchers for clothing from the Red Cross. And real British money again, no more dirty German Marks or "washers" (pfennigs). Life was good.

Branches of all His Majesty's Forces were billeted around and about. Wasn't it great getting back to the British way of life, driving and riding on the left of the road and seeing the Forces' vehicles. But, the sight we enjoyed and had a good laugh over, were the very old pre-war models that appeared on the roads, many that had been written off for scrap by the Germans, some still bore the word "scrot" painted on. These had been well hidden and cared for, they needed a good clean up and tuning and were rusted here and there, but, who cared? The "old-timers" were shown off with pride for they had escaped "Jerry's scrap yard".

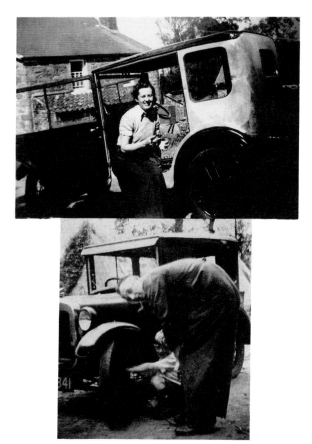

The Mouse Trap

The car I was proud to be driven around in was an Austin Seven, with a square back; it must have been an early '30's model. It was shabby but it ran well and I was the envy of many of the Nurses who christened that little car "The Mouse Trap". That little car had been well hidden in an old barn beneath an odd collection of old farm equipment.

No one refused lifts in the Mouse Trap, even Matron was pleased to have my boy friend run her around to various places, using it like a taxi. She went to the cinema quite a lot and he'd run her there whenever she wanted, much to the amusement of the Nursing Staff.

It was a treat to be able to visit the cinema again and to have films without a lot of propaganda in them. We began to realize how lucky we had been in many ways, seeing the news films of terrible bombings. At least we were never attacked in that way.

It was horrifying to see the films of the concentration camps, and the way those poor people were treated, also the terrifying Gas Chambers and the mounds of human skeletons stock-piled outside in the camps.

Oh, yes! We had a lot to be thankful for. Our suffering was nothing compared to the horrors of those camps.

The British lads were so happy to see the islanders enjoying life and lots of girls ready to make friends. And why not? The only thing is that one could not help noticing that those who had enjoyed the grey-green uniforms for 4-5 years were now <u>very</u> interested in the "Khaki". That's life!

The Nursing Staff were often invited to Forces "do's", dances or films. They always sent a general invite for a certain number of girls to make up their numbers. This way we were fortunate to meet different people and catch up with British life again.

They had their cinema at the Town Arsenal (Fire Station). Nursing staff who were off duty and wished to go to these films or dances were picked up from the hospital in jeeps. One evening some of the lads said it was a Frank Sinatra film on that night. "Who's Frank Sinatra?" The lads were so amazed that we had no idea who they meant. Would we <u>ever</u> catch up?

There were many incidents, some quite amusing, when we just didn't know what they were talking about. Those years of silence we had endured where the rest of the world was concerned was a lot of lost time, and so very very much had happened. There were new songs to learn, new dances, and different slang and expressions. We must have appeared to be quite daft at times. So much to learn about the war itself, some of which we had no idea had happened.

It was a beautiful sunny afternoon when an R.A.F. Jeep drove up just below the Children's Ward. We had some of the little patients all ready out on the balcony. Much to the children's surprise the R.A.F. boys came running up the fire escape asking the kids if they were ready to go. "Where?" and "What for?" They had no idea. It had all been arranged without them knowing a thing.

Another Nurse and I helped to get the patients comfortable and settled in the Jeep, then we accompanied them. I don't know who enjoyed the drive most, the kids or their carers!

We had an island tour and called in at the Airport, much to the delight of our boy burns patients. We were all entertained to tea and the kids had ice cream and "pop", which they weren't sure if they liked, they'd never to their knowledge had "pop" before. This was all partaken in the Jeep as we didn't wish to disturb any of them, but it didn't spoil any of the enjoyment.

The drive back to the hospital was fun, and we had a sing-song. I don't know quite what the officer and his driver thought but they were made to join in with the Nursery Rhymes. We all got back safe and sound, tired but happy, with no ill effects. It had been such great excitement for the kids.

They were full of the adventure for days. The 'planes they had seen, the long drive to get there, what they had had to eat and drink, the sing-song, to say nothing of their "great heroes", the R.A.F. personnel who had given them such a wonderful time. The Nurses enjoyed it too.

The two young boys with bad leg burns were transferred to the U.K. for treatment as soon as possible. Both returned to the island healed, but, unfortunately, somewhat disabled, having been bedridden and in splints for so long. They came back grown-up young men. One, sadly met with a fatal accident within a few years of his return. The other, I'm pleased to say, is running his own business and doing very well. May he continue so to do for a long time yet.

Many were the changes in those early days of Liberation. We had many official visits with regard to how we had coped over the years.

Sir Herbert Morrison from the Home Office and his entourage paid us a visit. He assessed everything and everybody. He went right through the whole establishment to see what essentials were needed.

Members of the Medical Corps spent a lot of time with us too, chatting and checking with patients and staff, asking many questions about our health and the diet we'd existed on. One officer suddenly asked: "Would you mind very much if I looked at your teeth? I'm a dental surgeon." Who were we to argue?

The patients were "tickled pink" to see their Nurses standing there in the middle of the ward with mouths wide open. Apparently he was very impressed to find our teeth in such good condition in spite of everything. Makes one think, doesn't it? We'd had no chocolate, no sweets or sugar, for a very long time.

Another officer was busy trying to explain the intricacies of the use of plasma, and about penicillin, things we'd never met before.

There was so much to learn again, so many different drugs and treatments that were all so very new to us.

We were appreciative of all the help we could get. It was great to meet fresh faces, someone different to work and converse with. Some Guernsey girls who had spent the war years in the U.K. had subsequently trained at various hospitals. They were among some of the first to arrive back to the island.

The important thing for them, I'm sure, was coming home to their relatives and friends, catching up on all the news and happenings of the past five years. We were very glad to have their help. They were rather surprised, sometimes alarmed, at our ways of working. What did they expect, we <u>were</u> five years behind the times.

But, from our point of view, we were rather amused by some of <u>them</u>, as there were many jobs that we did that they were quite unable to understand, let alone cope with. This made work all the more interesting and entertaining, and led to many discussions and comparing of notes and ways of working. In spite of their up-to-date ways, we were still able to show them a thing or two in the day-to-day running of the wards.

Another delightful surprise was when we met the four lovely Canadian Nurses, so smart in their St. John Ambulance Uniforms. They arrived in the island at the same time as Sir Herbert Morrison visited. We all felt very drab alongside these girls who were immaculate. They were so amused when we objected to standing near them in our worn and grubby-looking uniforms.

Before the war there was an advert. for "Persil soap Powder", which got clothes whiter than white. The illustrations always showed the "before and after" effect. We certainly felt and looked like the "befores" in our grey-white aprons alongside their dazzling white "afters".

The Canadians were enchanting girls and soon made many friends as they worked with us on the wards. They brought a lot of pleasure to the Nursing Staff to say nothing of the joy they brought to the patients, both male and female.

We learned so much from them regarding what had been going on in the world, which we had been shut away from for so long. Their help and friendship was greatly appreciated and we will for ever be grateful to their country for their help in saving us from starvation with those wonderful Red Cross Parcels.

Nov. 1945   TO OUR CANADIANS   C/O Clare Ogden
                                   A/S Pat Standish
                                   A/S Inis Moore
                                   A/S Alice Holland

When first we heard that Canadians would come
We knew they would find us slow and dumb,
We thought they'd show us the why's and wherefore's
And felt we would long to belt through the doors.
But now they are with us and have worked with us too
We feel that without them we never could do.
They've helped us and cheered us to such an extent
That we hope that they realize their time has been well spent.
They have found their way to each Sarnian's heart
In the Doctors' and Patients' and all Nursing Staff.
These girls are so great and we'll never forget
That to them and their country we owe a great debt.

                                                B.S.L.

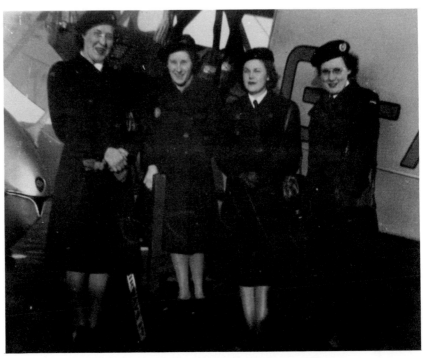

The Canadian St. John Ambulance Nurses

THE EVACUEES RETURN

Every day evacuees were returning to the island. Husbands who had been serving in H.M.'s Forces returned to the wives and children they'd left behind. Many children didn't know their fathers.

Then there were the wives who returned to husbands who had remained, either by choice or had been just too late to get off the island. The wives came back, often to find their husbands very weak and tired, but so happy to be together again.

Children who had evacuated with the schools came back to parents whom they didn't know or recognise. Many came back spoaking quite differently. Having spent those years in Scotland they spoke with a strong accent, and those who had lived in the North and Midlands of England spoke with many different dialects.

Nine and ten year olds came back as young adults, parents had missed out on the growing up years. Older children had grown up and started work, many had joined the forces and sadly many never returned.

Nothing was ever quite the same for those families. There was always that huge gap of five years when they were apart.

I was approached one morning in town a short time after Liberation, by a young man I had known before the war. He had evacuated and had served in the forces and was now back at his pre-war job. He asked if I would be willing to name girls who had fraternised with the Germans, as he knew I would probably know a lot about the "goings-on" through my work.

With some of his mates they were planning to expose these girls, and he did mention the shaving of heads and tar and feathers.

Well! I was so taken aback and explained that I would never pass on such information, that would be unethical. My work demanded confidentiality.

He was not very happy that I would in no way co-operate. But, as I told him at the time, I in no way endorsed all the fraternising, and that was my opinion. In any case, had he and his friends given a thought about what went on in the rest of the world during that time? Were all the British men perfect in their behaviour? Were there no girls of other nationalities willing to give comfort in various ways to our troops?

I did notice he had the grace to flush and was not looking me so straight in the eye. In no way did I wish to be involved and although I didn't condone a lot of the "goings-on", I told him I thought it best if he and his friends thought again.

Not having heard of any shaving or feathering, I hope a lot of embarrassment was saved. Those who did fraternise must have had their reasons and have to live with that for the rest of their lives.

We, who were here, saw a lot and knew a lot of what went on, but that is all water under the bridge now. Many were the stories of other happenings in the rest of the world. Who are we to judge?

There was so much to catch up on, after those years of restrictions and curfew. Friends and relatives to get in touch with on the other islands.

"The White Heather", an open fishing boat skippered by Mr. Zabiela, was one of the first to take passengers across to Sark, a favourite pre-war haunt of mine.

On a day off, we left the harbour in the morning with great anticipation of a good day's visit on Sark.

The trip was quite enjoyable. We were six passengers and two crew. My friend and I were sitting in the stern and caught quite a lot of spray, but found a small sail under the seat which gave ideal protection.

Much to our surprise, on board was another Nurse with her boy friend, and they too were longing to see Sark again. The other two passengers were two Jerseymen who were staying for a few days in Guernsey and they too wanted to see how Sark had fared.

By the time we arrived it was raining. We climbed the hill and were getting pretty wet. The other passengers had gone on their way and we two walked along the Avenue, past the shop, when a voice called out, "Nurse, Nurse is it really you?"

I looked around to see an ex-patient in the doorway. She was thrilled to see us. "Come in, come in, out of the rain." A typical Sark welcome. Before we knew it we were sitting in a cosy living room, drinking cups of tea and chatting of many things. The dear lady wanted us to stay for lunch, but when I explained we wished to visit some relatives of mine (whom she knew – everyone knows everyone on Sark) we were allowed to go on our way.

As it was my boy friend's first ever visit to Sark, I intended showing him as much as possible during the few hours we had. Off we set, trudging through the mud and slush, the roads were in a poor state, but it all added to the fun. My friend finished up with his trouser legs rolled up, looking as if he was going paddling. At least we saw the funny side of things, rain or no rain, and managed to cover quite a bit of the island.

We called in on the relatives to find out how they'd fared during the occupation. We were made very welcome, although we were in such a bedraggled state.

All too soon it was time to return to the boat. The rain had stopped, but there was quite a swell on the sea. Fortunately we were both very good sailors and quite enjoyed the trip back. The other four passengers were not so happy. My colleague and her boy friend and the two Jerseymen were looking very sorry for themselves.

The "Skipper" of the boat placed a large galvanised bucket in a very strategic position, knowing the seas would become much rougher once we left the shelter of the island.

The two of us were in the stern again, sheltering under the sail, eating chocolate and generally enjoying the rough trip, while the four others were passing the bucket around from one to the other. I suppose we were a bit mean, but we never let that Nurse forget about her Sark trip.

Later when we were both married, we kept in touch, and over the years often met up in Sark. We had many a laugh about the first Sark trip in an open boat just after Liberation.

Three or four months after Liberation we took another trip, this time to Jersey for a few days. We flew down and it took about fifteen minutes. A bit quicker and smoother than the Sark trip.

We wanted to see how Jersey had fared. We enjoyed the tours which included visits to various fortifications, also to their Underground Hospital which was most interesting. We also met up with our fellow passengers who had been on the Sark trip, having exchanged addresses. We had a pleasant evening and learnt about what had happened in Jersey. Much the same conditions as ours, the Jersey "crapaux" like the Guernsey "donkeys" enjoyed outwitting the enemy in so many little ways.

One story which has remained with me through the years is about a pig. The Jersey folk, like us, had to declare all animals and the Germans commandeered whatever meat they needed, often choosing one of the best animals. It was a difficult task to always keep one step ahead of "Jerry", but it was amazing what good ideas materialized when needed.

This was told to us by a Jersey cousin, a farmer. He, with a neighbouring farmer, had unlawfully slaughtered two of their pigs and someone somewhere had informed the Germans. One pig had been cut into joints, the other was still in carcass form.

On hearing the Germans were on their way to search the house, one farmer took baskets with pork joints out to the fields of cabbages and very quickly hid all the pieces under cabbages here and there, deep into the centre of the field.

Our farmer friend was in a predicament, how was he going to hide a full carcass? What could they do with it?

The Germans were on their way. They had finished searching the other farm and found nothing suspicious. They arrived and, in a somewhat aggressive manner, addressed the farmer. They started to search the farm and outbuildings, but found nothing. The whole family were doing their best to act as normally as possible with their day-to-day chores.

The officer-in-charge then ordered his men to search the house. When it came to searching the bedrooms, the farmer took the officer aside and explained that his mother was very ill, would they please try not to make too much noise in respect for the very sick old lady.

The Germans continued their search. When they came to the old lady's room, the farmer opened the door and invited the officer in. The officer took a quick look at the old lady and closed the door very quietly. Unknown to him at the time, and fortunately for the family, he was very close to "the dead pig". It was tucked up in bed with the old lady.

There we were all sitting in comfort, listening to their stories, the old lady, looking very fit and enjoying the story yet again. She told us she had never been so frightened in her life and that her fright must have made her very pale and short of breath. She never wanted to share her bed with a pig ever again. She was very proud of her son and the way he had outwitted the Germans. What a risk they took!

There are many stories of those days. Sadly we didn't think to record them at the time and so many have been forgotten.

GETTING BACK TO NORMAL

The town was beginning to look more attractive, with shops and businesses re-opening. Many small shops had kept going over the years with second-hand goods for sale. Islanders parted with a variety of goods to have money which enabled them to buy necessities.

Now all the new stocks appeared. The jewellers were doing very well as there was a rush of engagements and marriages. The hospital was a buzz of news, with such elation every day as news came of old friends and relatives returning.

Many of the staff became officially engaged, and, yes, I was happy to be in that number, but, as my fiancé happened to be a patient at the time, we just kept quiet about it. He had undergone surgery and I was on theatre duty for the operation.

We had exchanged rings just before he was admitted, unknown to any of the staff, which was difficult with us both working at the hospital. His ring was a little loose and it kept slipping off. The nurses on his ward kept joking about the lost ring in the bed, but didn't put two and two together. I kept my ring safely pinned <u>inside</u> my watch pocket, it was safe there.

The next thing I knew, I was transferred back on wards. Night duty on women's surgical. Rushing on duty one night, I was cornered by a colleague on the ward with me. "What's that I see?" she said. "Nothing", and I hastily turned away and popped the ring back into my pocket, trying to look very innocent and <u>very</u> busy.

"I saw a ring." − "You must be imagining things." − It was no good, the cat was out of the bag or should I say pocket. I asked her not to say anything to anyone, and we got on with our job. At 4 a.m. we usually had a cup of tea and a snack before waking the patients at 5 a.m. Just before 4 a.m. Staff Nurse asked if I'd do her a favour and sort the dressing trays for her, for the morning treatments, which I willingly did.

When I went back to the duty room for my cup of tea, the table was laid with quite a spread and sitting at the head of the table was my fiancé, all dressed up in his dressing gown and slippers with a big grin on his face. Staff Nurse had been over to men's ward, got him up out of bed and brought him over to have tea with us as a bit of a celebration. It was very sweet of the girls to have gone to so much trouble, and we did appreciate their kindness, even at 4 o'clock in the morning.

Of course, when it came time to awaken the patients most of those ladies were already awake wanting to know what all the whispering and giggling was about, and the one nearest the duty room insisted that she had heard a man's voice. It was no good denying anything any more. Our secret was out. All the night staff knew and it didn't take long for the day staff to hear too.

Later that morning after report, on going off-duty, who should I meet but Matron. "Nurse! What's this I hear? − You know very well that had I known what I know now, you would never have been allowed in that theatre when John had his operation."

"Yes, Matron, I know. I'm very sorry."

However, she wished us all the best and we were forgiven. About eleven months later she made our day by being a guest at our wedding.

It does not seem possible that all this occurred fifty years ago.

To any of my old colleagues who may have read these anecdotes, I hope they have brought back many happy memories.

Sadly many of our old friends are no longer with us, but, I know those of us still around remember them with affection.

THE END

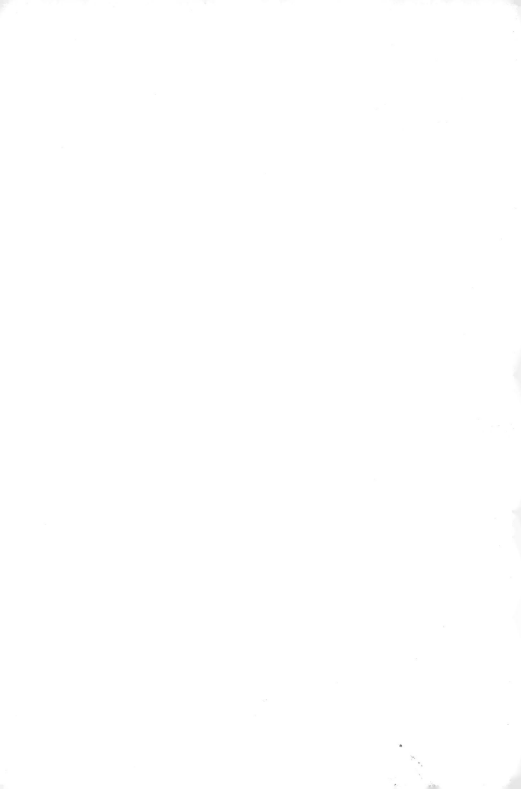